OUTPATIENT MEDICINE RECALL

RECALL SERIES EDITOR

LORNE H. BLACKBOURNE, M.D.
General Surgeon
Major, Medical Corps
United States Army
Fort Eustis, Virginia

OUTPATIENT MEDICINE RECALL

SENIOR EDITOR

JOHN P. FRANKO, M.D.
Assistant Professor of Clinical Family Medicine
University of Virginia Health Sciences Center
Charlottesville, Virginia

ASSISTANT EDITOR

STEVEN A. MEIXEL, M.D.
Professor of Clinical Family Medicine
University of Virginia Health Sciences Center
Charlottesville, Virginia

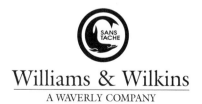

Williams & Wilkins
A WAVERLY COMPANY

BALTIMORE • PHILADELPHIA • LONDON • PARIS • BANGKOK
BUENOS AIRES • HONG KONG • MUNICH • SYDNEY • TOKYO • WROCLAW

Editor: Elizabeth Nieginski
Manager, Development Editing: Julie P. Scardiglia
Managing Editor: Darrin Kiessling
Marketing Manager: Rebecca Himmelheber
Development Editor: Rosanne Hallowell
Production Coordinator: Felecia R. Weber
Designer: Karen Klinedinst
Illustration Planner: Felecia R. Weber
Cover Designer: Karen Klinedinst
Typesetter: Maryland Composition Co., Inc.
Printer/Binder: RR Donnelley & Sons Company

Copyright © 1998 Williams & Wilkins

351 West Camden Street
Baltimore, Maryland 21201-2436 USA

Rose Tree Corporate Center
1400 North Providence Road
Building II, Suite 5025
Media, Pennsylvania 19063-2043 USA

Accurate indications, adverse reactions and dosage schedules for drugs are provided in this book, but it is possible that they may change. The reader is urged to review the package information data of the manufacturers of the medications mentioned.

Printed in the United States of America

Library of Congress Cataloging-in-Publication Data

Outpatient medicine recall / senior editor, John P. Franko : assistant
   editor, Steven A. Meixel.
     p.   cm.
   Includes index.
   ISBN 0-683-18018-5
   1. Ambulatory medical care—Examinations, questions, etc.
  I. Franko, John P. II. Meixel, Steven A.
   [DNLM: 1. Ambulatory Care—examination questions. 2. Family
Practice—examination questions. WB 18.2 094 1998]
RC58.087   1998
616′.0076—dc21
DNLM/DLC
for Library of Congress   97-34982
                                    CIP

To purchase additional copies of this book, call our customer service department at **(800) 638-0672** or fax orders to **(800) 447-8438**. For other book services, including chapter reprints and large quantity sales, ask for the Special Sales department.

Canadian customers should call **(800) 665-1148**, or fax **(800) 665-0103**. For all other calls originating outside of the United States, please call **(410) 528-4223** or fax us at **(410) 528-8550**.

Visit Williams & Wilkins on the Internet: http://www.wwilkins.com or contact our customer service department at **custserv@wwilkins.com**. Williams & Wilkins customer service representatives are available from 8:30 am to 6:00 pm, EST, Monday through Friday, for telephone access.

98 99 00
1 2 3 4 5 6 7 8 9 10

This book is dedicated to:

My parents, Bernard and Marie, who showed me that all things are possible with hard work and love . . .

My siblings, who never let me forget who I am and where I came from . . .

My colleagues, friends, and patients in Danville and Charlottesville, Virginia, who, over the years, helped me acquire the information that is found in this book . . .

B. Lewis Barnett, Jr., M.D., and Michael Coates, M.D., who gave me the opportunity of a lifetime . . .

My children, Erin, John, Jr., and Lisa, who have shown their patience and love throughout this project and are my joy and inspiration . . .

Especially my wife, Barb, who tolerates my moods each day, is my partner in everything that I do, and is the love of my life.

Contents

Contributors

David C. Slawson, M.D.
Associate Professor of Clinical Family Medicine
University of Virginia Health Sciences Center
Charlottesville, Virginia

Richard A. VanMeter, M.D.
Family Medicine Resident
University of Virginia Health Sciences Center
Charlottesville, Virginia

Elizabeth K. Buchinski, M.D.
Practicing Physician
Manassas, Virginia

Jeffrey M. Feit, M.D.
Family Medicine Resident
University of Virginia Health Sciences Center
Charlottesville, Virginia

Kavian Milani, M.D.
Family Medicine Resident
University of Virginia Health Sciences Center
Charlottesville, Virginia

Preface

Outpatient Medicine Recall is a continuation of the Recall series initiated by the Department of Surgery at the University of Virginia. Since rotations in Outpatient Medicine are relatively new at the University of Virginia, we did not have an unofficial written tradition of medical student information to draw on as this text was developed, as was the case for *Surgical Recall*. Therefore, all questions were developed by faculty and residents in the University of Virginia Department of Family Medicine. We anticipate that the content will be helpful for medical students and other persons learning primary care medicine.

1   Introduction

USING THE STUDY GUIDE

This study guide is designed to help you learn the basic concepts that you will be tested on during your clinical clerkship in Ambulatory Medicine or Family Practice. The question-and-answer format is used to help you study for verbal and/or written tests. The content focuses on the basic information you need for a foundation on which you can build further knowledge. This guide does not cover every topic in Ambulatory Medicine, nor does it cover every aspect of the topics covered. You are encouraged to use textbooks to learn the less common aspects of common problems as well as less common problems.

    The other goal of this guide is to help you when you are actually seeing patients in the outpatient setting. Using this guide in the clinical setting will help you obtain appropriate information from patients as you interview them, prepare concise presentations with relevant facts, and write outpatient notes and prescriptions. Good luck, and enjoy your outpatient experience.

OUTPATIENT NOTES

The outpatient note, as with all medical records, is both a medical and legal document. The medical information must be precise and complete, so that the next person who reads the record understands the relevant issues, the diagnosis, the treatment, and follow-up plan. The legal implications of the record are twofold. First, it is used as evidence if it is needed in a criminal or civil case involving the patient. These cases can involve the state (in a criminal case), another individual or corporation (if your patient decides to sue over injuries obtained in an accident), or you (in a malpractice case). Second, the record documents the level of service provided and, therefore, documents whether the charge submitted to the insurance carrier is appropriate. In all of these situations, it is important that the record is legible and complete. Errors should be crossed out with one line, and then initialed and dated. Never scribble through an entry. If your handwriting is poor, print legibly. It is difficult (and sometimes embarrassing) to try to use or defend an illegible record in court.

    The outpatient clinic (office) note contains the same elements as an inpatient note.

It is organized in the "SOAP" format:

S is for **subjective.** All historical information is contained in this section. The note should begin with a concise statement of the chief complaint followed by all relevant positives and negatives regarding the history of present illness, past medical history (including medical problems, past surgeries, medications and allergies), social history, family history, and review of systems.

O is for **objective.** Vital signs, physical findings, labs, radiographs, and all other objective data are included in this section.

A *is for* **assessment** and *P* is for **plan.** These elements are combined in a problem-oriented record so that each assessment is listed and numbered, and the treatment plan is recorded in the same heading. Each office or clinic will have some variation on this theme. You should ask what format is used during your orientation in each clinic. Remember:

1. You are a transient member of the clinical staff, so always document information in a manner that can be understood by the next person to read the chart.
2. Write legibly.
3. Record in the *plan* section of your note the dosages, quantities, and refills of prescribed medications, particularly for controlled substances. Also include OTC medication recommendations.
4. Always include instructions for follow-up. Never use *follow-up p.r.n.*. Explain to the patient the details about what constitutes worsening of the present problem and record it in the chart. Instruct the patient to return for the next health maintenance evaluation if follow-up is not needed for the presenting problem.
5. Review your outpatient note with your supervisor, and ask for feedback.

WRITING PRESCRIPTIONS

Writing prescriptions is simple, but different than ordering medication for a hospitalized patient. The prescription form varies slightly from state to state, but it usually has areas for writing in the patient's name and address, number of refills, DEA number, and whether or not voluntary formulary (generic) substitution is allowed. Look at the prescription pad in the office or clinic where you are working and become familiar with the format. Students (MD, DO, NP, PA) should always make sure that a licensed physician signs the prescription before they or the physician gives it to the patient.

The largest area of the prescription form is blank, and it is where you write the medication order. The order is comprised of three parts:

1. **Medication, dosage, and formulation.** You need to be certain that the dosages (e.g., mg, g) and formulations (e.g., tablets, pills, suspension, cream) are consistent with those supplied by manufacturers. Check the "How Supplied" section of the *PDR* or other similar references. Nonstandard dosages or formulations can be ordered but are expensive to prepare; the pharmacist will usually call to verify these orders.

2. **Quantity dispensed.** The number symbol (#) is frequently used, followed by the number of pills or capsules for the patient. For liquid or semisolid medications (e.g., creams, lotions, ointments), write the amount to be dispensed in volume or weight units (e.g., ml, fl oz, g, oz).
3. **Instructions for use (Sig).** Write instructions for how many, how often, and by which route the patient should take the medication. These instructions should be clear, concise, and simple. They are printed on the bottle or container, and the patient uses these instructions as a guide to taking the medication. Many symbols and abbreviations can be used to decrease the amount of writing required. Many of these shortcuts were derived from Latin.

PRESCRIPTION EXAMPLES

A 45-year-old man has sinusitis. You decide he needs amoxicillin three times each day for 2 weeks. The prescription should read as follows:

Amoxicillin 500 mg

42

Sig: Take one tid for 2 weeks

No refills

A 1-year-old child has otitis media. You decide to treat her with amoxicillin 30 mg/kg/day, divided three times each day. She weighs 12.5 kg.

Amoxicillin suspension 125 mg/5 ml

Dispense 150 ml

Sig: Take one teaspoon po tid for 10 days

No refills

A 65-year-old woman with stable hypertension needs a refill for her diuretic. You plan to see her in 6 months.

HCTZ 25-mg tablets

100

Sig: Take one po qd

One refill

A 23-year-old man has tinea corporis on the skin of his abdomen. You decide to treat him with ketoconazole cream for 2 weeks.

Ketoconazole cream

Dispense 15 g

Sig: Apply to the affected area bid for 2 weeks

One refill

INTERVIEWING PATIENTS

The following pointers are to remind you of important issues involved in interviewing patients. They should also help you review strategies for dealing with potentially difficult patient dynamics that you will encounter in outpatient practice.

HELPFUL HINTS

First and foremost, **LISTEN.** If you are too involved trying to think of the next question you want to ask, you will miss most of the information the patient is trying to give you.

Sit at or below the patient's level. It is a less dominating position, and it will help the patient to relax and feel more in control.

Maintain comfortable eye contact. Don't stare into the patient's eyes and don't avoid eye contact.

Look for the unspoken message. Patients often have a hidden agenda for coming to the office. Pay attention to body language, facial expressions, voice intonation, and other nonverbal cues. Ask open-ended questions, and allow the patient to help lead the conversation so that you avoid missing the real reason that the patient came to the office. **Frequently repeat to the patient a synopsis of what you thought you heard the patient say.** This synopsis reassures the patient that you are really listening and gives them a chance to make corrections and/or additions to your interpretation of the information.

Never ignore the "Just one more thing, doctor . . . " or "By the way . . . " phrases as you are headed out the door for what you thought was a completed encounter. This means that, despite your best efforts, you did not address the real reason that the patient came to the office. This final statement is frequently the most important information that the patient will give you.

PATIENT ENCOUNTERS WITH ATYPICAL DYNAMICS

Most patient encounters are straightforward, pleasant, and greatly enhanced by your involvement as a student doctor. However, some patients experience anxiety about the loss of control they feel during an encounter with a physician. Some patients are unable to negotiate control of the relationship and/or encounter with their physician (and this is usually because the physician refuses to allow the patient any control). And, some patients have personality traits that make these negotiations anxiety provoking and difficult. These patients often develop communication strategies that make the physician–patient encounter more challenging. The patient uses these strategies to attempt to alter the dynamic of the encounter and/or relationship, so that he/she feels more control. Instead of wrestling for control, always try to work with the patient in a reassuring manner. The following examples describe some of the more frequently encountered strategies.

The Passive–Aggressive Patient

This passive–aggressive patient will be one of your greatest challenges as a student doctor. This patient often finds flaws in your statements that, while not contradicting you directly, will increase your feelings of inadequacy. Also, you can rarely satisfy all of this patient's complaints, no matter how hard you try. This dynamic can lead to unsatisfactory encounters and may tempt you to take a more authoritarian tone with the patient in an escalating attempt to show that you really do have the answer. This approach will make things worse.

Remember, passive–aggressiveness is a patient's attempt to gain control of the situation. Maintain an honest and open attitude. Acknowledge past treatment failures. Allow the patient to lead the focus of the interview as much as possible. Giving the patient more direct control often helps the patient feel more comfortable and have less need to be passive–aggressive.

The Manipulative Patient

Manipulative patients have specific goals and/or treatment expectations, and they attempt to use medical symptoms to manipulate you into satisfying their expectations. Expect great praise if you satisfy their expectations and great criticism if you do not. A good example of this patient type is the drug-seeking patient.

During the encounter remain calm, open, and direct. Try not to feed into the emotional escalation that often occurs if their demands are not met. Patiently develop a reasonable approach to their problem, and state positively what you can do for them and what you cannot. Avoid making exceptions to previously stated limitations. Consistency in approach is important in managing these patients. Input from their primary physician can be invaluable.

The Dependent Patient

Dependent patients initially seem pleasant and rewarding. They will tell you what a wonderful physician you are and how much you have helped them. However, as time goes by, symptoms persist despite extensive evaluation and multiple therapies. The patient will call or come to the office frequently and sometimes begin to call you at home. They rely on you to "make them well" and expect you to explain every symptom that they might experience even transiently.

When you begin to feel the weight of the dependent patient's demands, your first instinct may be to try to see them as infrequently as possible. Avoid this temptation, because it usually leads to an escalation of symptoms that forces you to see them.

See the patient frequently but set limits on the amount of time for the encounter and enforce them strictly. This reassures the patient as to your availability and interest. Use your influence to help the patient take small steps toward being more self-reliant. Counseling can help the patient deal with underlying self-esteem and confidence issues.

The Hostile Patient

Remain calm, and don't take the patient's hostility personally. Comment on the process (e.g., "You seem angry; would you like to talk about it?" or "You seem angry, is there something that I said that upset you?") Be open and allow the patient to vent their feelings, as long as it is in a nonthreatening manner. Answer questions honestly, and acknowledge valid grievances. This is not a time for feeble excuses or to "shoot from the hip." If you feel physically threatened, leave the room.

The Seductive Patient

Sexual advances from a patient may be subtle, direct, or somewhere in between. A sexual advance, especially from a patient you find attractive, can be ego gratifying and tempting. Remember, is *always* unethical to use the physician–patient relationship to initiate a romantic or sexual relationship with a patient. In addition, you risk losing your medical license and being charged with sexual harassment. It is best never to become romantically involved with a patient.

If you feel that a patient is making attempts to be seductive, maintain a professional demeanor and do not encourage or return the remarks. If the patient is more direct, then you need to be more direct in your response to discourage further advances. It is important to have a nurse chaperone for the entire physical examination and consider a chaperone for the history as well. Refer the patient to another physician if the advances continue despite your best efforts to discourage the behavior.

2 ___

Common Office Procedures

ELECTROCARDIOGRAM (EKG)

What is it?

A graphic recording of the electrical activity of the heart; it measures the direction, magnitude, and duration of electrical forces at 12 points in two planes (six vertical and six horizontal)

How is it performed?

Leads are attached to gel-coated pads, which are placed on the extremities and across the chest.

Where are the limb leads placed?

The four limb leads are attached to the forearms and lower legs. The limb leads are color coded and labeled: RA (right arm), LA (left arm), RL (right leg) and LL (left leg).

Where are the chest leads placed?

The chest leads are numbered 1 through 6. Lead 1 is placed at the fourth right intercostal space adjacent to the sternum; lead 2 is placed at the fourth left intercostal space adjacent to the sternum; lead 4 is placed at the fifth left intercostal space in the midclavicular line; lead 3 is placed midway between leads 2 and 4; lead 5 is placed at the sixth left intercostal space in the anterior axillary line; and lead 6 is placed at the sixth left intercostal space in the midaxillary line.

What should be the EKG paper speed?

Most modern EKG machines are run with the touch of a button to get a 12-lead EKG. The paper speed should be 25 mm/sec, with vertical deflection set at 10 mm/mv.

What are the indications for an EKG?

The EKG is used most commonly to evaluate cardiac problems, some of the most common being arrhythmias, ischemia, pericarditis, and hypertension (to detect LVH). Some metabolic abnormalities (e.g., hypo- or hyperkalemia) and toxic drug level effects (e.g., procainamide) can also be detected with the EKG.

Helpful hints

1. The EKG is **NOT** indicated as a routine screening test in otherwise healthy, asymptomatic persons.
2. Incorrect lead placement or settings of the EKG machine may cause unusual or bizarre tracings. If the EKG looks unusual, check lead placement and machine settings.

CRYOTHERAPY

What is it?

The use of liquid gas to induce a controlled frostbite injury to abnormal tissue in order to destroy it

How is it performed?

By directly (open system) or indirectly (closed system) applying the liquid gas (usually nitrogen or carbon dioxide) to skin or other epithelial tissue allowing the tissue to freeze. The freeze is maintained for a predetermined time period, depending on the type of lesion and location. The tissue is allowed to thaw completely and then frozen a second time.

What is it used for?

Destruction of benign skin lesions (e.g., warts, skin tags, actinic keratoses) and low-grade neoplasms of the uterine cervix

Helpful hints

1. NEVER freeze a suspected malignant skin lesion (especially a pigmented lesion) or high-grade neoplasm of the cervix. It could result in incomplete destruction of the lesion, leading to delayed diagnosis, staging, and treatment of the malignancy.

2. Cryotherapy is more effective on lesions with a high water content. Therefore, skin lesions should be soaked in water for 5 – 10 minutes before treatment.
3. Indirect (closed) systems ("guns") can have uneven thermal transfer. This is minimized if a thin layer of a water-based lubricant is placed on the applicator tip before freezing the lesion.

FECAL OCCULT BLOOD TESTING

What is it?	One of several commercially available chemical tests to evaluate feces for the presence of small quantities of blood
How is it performed?	Feces collected from either a bowel movement or rectal exam are placed on the test card and a chemical developer is added. A color change occurs if blood (or other reducing substances) is present in sufficient quantities.
What is it used for?	1. To detect blood loss from the GI tract in patients with signs and/or symptoms of GI disease (e.g., peptic ulcer disease, diverticular disease, inflammatory bowel disease) that could induce blood loss 2. Screening test for colon and/or rectal polyps and/or cancer
Helpful hints	1. Restrict foods high in reducing substances (e.g., red meat, vitamin C) before testing to make the test more accurate. 2. Rehydration of samples sent in by patients from home is not recommended. This increases false positives.

HEMATOCRIT (HCT)

What is it?	The percent volume of whole blood occupied by red blood cells

How is it measured?
Blood obtained by fingerstick (capillary hct) or phlebotomy (central hct) is placed in a capillary tube, and one end is sealed with clay. The capillary tube is centrifuged at high speed to separate the cells from the serum. The hct is the length of the column of red cells divided by the length of the entire column of cells and serum multiplied by 100 and expressed in units of volume percent. This calculation can be done by direct measurement of the tube or by using one of many commercial devices available.

What is it used for?
The hct is used to evaluate the severity of blood loss in patients with signs or symptoms of acute or chronic blood loss.

What is another name for low hct?
Anemia

Why is hct an indirect measure of nutrition?
Because normal red cell metabolism depends on the ingestion, absorption, and metabolism of several common nutrients, such as iron, folic acid, and vitamin B_{12}. Many other medical conditions can affect the production of red blood cells and result in anemia.

INTRAMUSCULAR (IM) INJECTION

What is it?
A technique of administering pharmaceuticals to a patient that bypasses the GI tract (parenteral administration)

How is it performed?
The skin over the injection site is cleansed with alcohol and allowed to dry. A thin gauge (ga) needle is placed on the syringe containing the medication and inserted through the cleansed skin into the underlying muscle. Negative pressure is applied to the plunger of the syringe and the hub of the needle is examined for a flashback of blood. If no blood is seen, it is safe to inject the medication into the muscle.

Why would blood flash back into the hub of the needle or syringe?

The needle is likely in the lumen of a blood vessel, and the medication should not be injected. The needle should be repositioned and the procedure repeated. If no blood flashes back, it is safe to inject.

What is it used for?

Administration of pharmaceuticals (e.g., medications, immunizations) that cannot or should not be given orally; it may also be used to obtain a higher peak serum level of medications than can be obtained with oral administration (e.g., antibiotics for serious infections). Agents cannot be given orally if the patient has nausea, vomiting, or other GI problems that make it improbable that the medication will be retained in the GI tract or be properly absorbed. Some agents (e.g., most immunizations) cannot survive in a biologically active form if exposed to the low gastric pH and must be administered intramuscularly.

Should you use the same needle for drawing the medication into the needle and administering the medication?

No. Change the needle after drawing up the medication to avoid irritation or contamination of the skin and/or subcutaneous tissue with the medication.

How long should the needle be?

Long enough to reach into the body of the muscle. The subcutaneous fat layer can be very thick or almost nonexistent. Injection of the pharmaceutical into the subcutaneous fat or in deep soft tissues outside of the muscle can cause potentially serious complications and/or alter the absorption of the agent.

Helpful hints

1. Used needles and some pharmaceuticals are biohazards, and some pharmaceuticals are toxic waste. Always dispose of used materials properly.
2. When possible, instruct the patient to relax the muscle before inserting the needle. This will result in less trauma and pain.
3. Always report needlestick accidents.

JOINT ASPIRATION/INJECTION

What is it?

Procedure used to obtain a sample of synovial fluid from a joint and/or inject medication into a joint

How is it performed?

The involved joint is examined, and approach into the joint is chosen. Strict sterile preparation and technique are followed including skin preparation, draping, sterile gloves, sterile needles, and sterile syringes. The skin and injection tract are anesthetized by local infiltration with anesthetic, such as lidocaine, using a narrow-gauge needle (25–27 ga). A large needle (18–20 ga) is attached to a 10–20 ml syringe, passed through the anesthetized tract into the joint, and synovial fluid is aspirated and/or medication injected.

What is it used for?

1. Synovial fluid is evaluated to determine the etiology of joint pain or effusion.
2. Medication is injected to relieve joint pain and/or inflammation.

Helpful hints

1. Synovial fluid is very viscous, so a large-gauge needle is required to aspirate synovial fluid.
2. Obtain synovial fluid before injecting any type of medication into the joint. Foreign substances will preclude valid synovial fluid analysis.
3. Injection of steroids into a joint can cause a delayed chemical irritation in the joint. Warn the patient that the joint may get worse before it gets better.

KOH (POTASSIUM HYDROXIDE) PREP

What is it?

A method used to identify fungal elements in epithelial tissues.

How is it performed?

A sample of epithelium (e.g., scrapings of skin, scalp, or nails; vaginal secretions collected with a cotton-tipped swab) is placed on a clean microscope slide. Two drops of KOH solution are placed on the sample and mixed with the epithelial sample and a coverslip placed over the mixture. It can be gently heated by passing it over an alcohol lamp flame two or three times; or it can sit for several minutes to allow the KOH to lyse the epithelial cells, so that fungal elements are more easily identified. The specimen is then examined under the high/dry power of a microscope for fungal elements (buds and hyphae).

Helpful hints

1. Fungi are normal skin flora. Presence of fungal elements is strongly suggestive of fungal infection but not necessarily diagnostic.
2. KOH prep can show the presence of yeast and fungi but it cannot identify the exact organisms.
3. When evaluating vaginal secretions, always look at the saline prep first. This gives the KOH time to lyse cells and will help identify trichomonads, because their motility decreases with cooling and drying outside the vagina.

PAPANICOLAOU SMEAR (PAP SMEAR)

What is it?

A cytologic screening test used to detect cancerous and precancerous lesions of the uterine cervix; a sample of cells scraped from the outside of the cervix is examined.

How is it done?

The cervix is visualized using a vaginal speculum. The speculum can be warmed and lubricated with water only; other lubricants alter the cell structure, making interpretation impossible. A sample of squamous and columnar epithelial cells and cells from the transition zone (T zone) between the squamous and columnar cells is obtained by scraping these areas with one or more collection devices (e.g., spatula and cytobrush or one of the endo- and ectocervical combination brushes). The sample is then smeared on a microscope slide, promptly preserved by applying a fixing agent to prevent cellular artifact from drying, and sent to the pathology lab for evaluation and interpretation.

When is it used?

The Pap smear is part of the health maintenance evaluation for women. The Pap smear should be included in a woman's evaluation when she becomes sexually active. It should be performed yearly for 3 consecutive years and, if normal each time, can be performed every 3 years thereafter, as long as the woman remains in the low-risk group and the Pap smears remain normal. Higher risk groups [e.g., those with multiple sexual partners, those having unprotected intercourse outside a mutually monogamous relationship, history of sexually transmitted disease (especially HPV), previous minor abnormalities on Pap smear] should be screened yearly. Highest risk groups (e.g., those with HIV/AIDS or with recent mild-to-moderate abnormalities on Pap smear) should be screened more often; exact frequency recommended varies depending on source.

Helpful hints

1. Be familiar with the collection device used in the clinic or office you are working in—specifically, how the device should be applied to the cervix and how many rotations it takes to obtain an optimum sample.
2. Consider postponing the Pap smear if the woman has clinical evidence of vaginitis or cervicitis. Treat infection and have the woman return in 10–12 weeks for Pap.
3. Menstruation can also interfere with interpretation of the Pap smear, so

have the patient reschedule her exam in 2–3 weeks.
4. If possible, the woman should avoid introduction of anything into the vagina (e.g., douche, spermicide, having intercourse) 24 hours before the Pap.

PEAK EXPIRATORY FLOW

What is it?

Measurement of the maximum expiratory volume per unit time (liters per minute) that an individual can produce during an intense forced expiratory effort

How is it measured?

Place a disposable mouthpiece on a peak flowmeter, and place the flow indicator at zero. Carefully instruct the patient to take a deep breath and then exhale into the mouthpiece as quickly and forcefully as possible. The indicator will move with airflow; you should read the number at the level of the indicator. This number is the peak expiratory flow in liters per minute for that exhalation. Compare the reading with the patient's previous best peak flows or with standardized tables of normal values to determine the patient's performance.

What is it used for?

Peak flow measurements are used to assess the severity of reactive airways disease (e.g., asthma, COPD). It can be used in the acute situation for patients with worsening symptoms to objectively measure the severity of the impairment of airflow, which can help guide therapy. It can also be used to follow asymptomatic or minimally symptomatic patients with chronic asthma to objectively measure effectiveness of maintenance therapy and/or identify when further treatment is needed.

Helpful hints

1. Patients who have never used the peak flowmeter usually need careful

instruction and several practice attempts to learn proper technique. Be sure the meter is held properly; the patient should not interfere with the movement of the flow indicator (pointer) or obstruct the exhaust openings.

2. A single peak flowmeter has good reproducibility from measurement to measurement, but there can be significant variability from meter to meter; therefore, it is important for the patient to use a single meter for all measurements (i.e., patients should have their own meter and bring it to the office for all visits related to their obstructive airways disease).

SALINE (WET) PREP

What is it?

A method used to examine vaginal secretions to evaluate for two of the etiologies of vaginitis

How is it performed?

A sample of vaginal secretions (discharge) is collected on a cotton-tipped swab and smeared on a clean microscope slide. One to two drops of normal saline are placed on the sample, a coverslip is placed, and the sample/saline mixture is examined under the high/dry power of the microscope.

What three things should the slide examiner look for?

1. First, **look for movement of flagellated organisms.** The movement is jerky and intermittent (as opposed to the smooth flow of brownian movement) and can be seen under medium or high/ dry power. The head of the organism is about the size of a WBC. These organisms are trichomonads, are sexually transmitted, and cause marked vaginal inflammation (many WBCs).

2. Next, **look for clue cells.** These are epithelial cells that appear coated with round dots (inclusions) that often obscure the outer edge of the cell membrane. The inclusions are anaerobic cocci that have replaced the normal vaginal flora resulting in vaginal discharge. Clue cells are diagnostic of bacterial vaginosis.

3. Finally, **look for WBCs.** More than 30 WBCs per high-powered field indicate significant vaginal inflammation and a cause needs to be identified.

Helpful hints

1. Examine the specimen ASAP after collection. Cooling and/or drying can render the trichomonads immotile, making them difficult or impossible to identify.

2. Bacterial vaginosis can be present without significant inflammation. If a woman has vaginal discharge but no WBCs, look closely for clue cells. Bacterial vaginosis is also a cause of preterm labor and should be treated, if found, in pregnant women.

3. Wet prep can also be done on a swab of the cervix. More than 10 WBCs per high-powered field suggest cervicitis.

TUBERCULOSIS SKIN TEST (PPD)

What is it?

A diagnostic test to evaluate if a person has had an infection with *Mycobacterium tuberculosis*

How is it done?

0.1 ml of a 5TU (tuberculin units/0.1 ml) solution of a purified protein derivative of *M. tuberculosis* is injected **intradermally** (usually in the skin of the volar aspect of the forearm). If bleeding occurs at the injection site, the injection was too deep.

What are we looking for?

Induration (palpable swelling) of the skin 48-72 hours after injection. Induration with a diameter of 15 mm is considered a positive reaction in all cases. There are high risk and/or immunocompromised conditions (e.g., immigrants from countries with high endemic infection rates, HIV/AIDS, certain cancers) in which induration of less than 15 mm may indicate a positive test.

Helpful hints

1. Be sure to measure induration, not erythema (redness). There is usually a large area of erythema around the indurated portion of the reaction.
2. Measure the largest diameter of induration.

TYMPANOMETRY

What is it?

A test that measures the mobility of the tympanic membrane (TM)

How is it performed?

The tympanometer, with a large earpiece attached, is placed in the ear canal, totally occluding and sealing it. The tympanometer is activated while the seal of the ear canal is maintained with firm but gentle pressure on the handle of the tympanometer. The tympanometer generates a gradual increase followed by a gradual decrease in the pressure in the external auditory canal (EAC) and measures the movement of the TM secondary to the pressure in the EAC. The machine then prints a graph depicting the movement of the TM with change in pressure.

What is it used for?

Tympanometry evaluates for abnormalities of the middle ear and TM. The most common abnormalities of the middle ear are related to infection and subsequent effusions. Tympanometry detects the effusions as decreases in TM mobility. Because fluid is not compressible, the TM is less mobile if an effusion is present and the TM is shown

to be less mobile on tympanometry.
Also, if the TM is perforated, it will not
move, even with changing pressures.

Helpful hints

1. Visualize the TM just before
   tympanometry. Wax or other
   materials occluding the EAC can
   produce invalid results.
2. Maintain a good seal of the EAC for
   an accurate measurement.

URINALYSIS

What is it?

Evaluation of urine using chemical and/
or microscopic techniques

What is the chemical technique?

Dipstick urinalysis

How does it work?

The dipstick is a plastic strip that has
one or more chemically impregnated
pads attached. It is dipped in a freshly
collected urine specimen and color
changes of each pad are compared with
standards on a chart, usually on the label
of the container containing the dipsticks.
The color change comparisons are made
at the appropriate time intervals
described for each test on the label.

What do these tests evaluate?

Some of the common tests evaluate the
urine for protein, glucose, RBCs,
bilirubin, nitrites, leukocyte esterase,
specific gravity, and pH.

What are the microscopic techniques?

8–10 ml of fresh urine are placed in a
test tube and centrifuged for 5 minutes.
All but about 1 ml of supernatant is
discarded, and the sediment is
resuspended in the 1 cc of supernatant.
One drop of this suspension is placed on
a microscope slide and covered with a
coverslip. The specimen is then
examined under the high/dry power of
the microscope for cells, bacteria,
crystals, and casts. Type and average
number of each component per high
power field are noted and recorded.

What is urinalysis used for?

It is used to help evaluate for urinary tract infection, metabolic disease (e.g., diabetes, dehydration, biliary disease), renal parenchymal disease (e.g., nephritis, nephrosis), and renal excretory abnormalities (e.g., calculus formation).

Helpful hints

1. Presence of more than a few squamous epithelial cells indicates contamination of the specimen from the perineum, vagina, and/or rectum.
2. Save about 3 ml of urine in a separate container before using the dipstick so that an accurate culture is obtained, if needed (the dipstick is not sterile and can introduce bacteria into the specimen).
3. Urinalysis is usually not recommended as a screening test in asymptomatic, low-risk patients (pregnancy is an exception to this rule).

URINE β HUMAN CHORIONIC GONADOTROPIN (βHCG)

What is it?

Antibody test that detects βHCG in urine

What is it used for?

Presence of detectable levels of βHCG in urine indicates pregnancy

How is it performed?

Urine is placed on a material impregnated with antibodies to βHCG. A solution is added that causes a color change if antigen–antibody complexes are present. A positive test has a colored line or a + sign and a negative test has no color change or a − sign, depending on the test manufacturer.

What time of day is best for specimen collection?

The first-voided morning specimen contains the highest levels of βHCG and is the most sensitive specimen to use to detect pregnancy.

How soon after conception can the test detect βHCG in urine?

The commercially available assays used in medical offices are very sensitive and can detect βHCG in urine as soon as 6 days after conception. This is only 1 to 2 days after serum βHCG levels can be detected.

What may interfere with the test?

Large amounts of blood and debris can interfere with the assay. Centrifuge the urine before testing if a large amount of sediment is present.

3

Common Presenting Symptoms

This chapter briefly reviews some of the most common general presenting symptoms. The goal of this chapter is to give you a "place to start" when seeing patients in the ambulatory setting. These lists of differential diagnoses are not intended to be complete, but they include the most common problems seen in the outpatient setting. Most of these problems are also covered in more detail in later chapters.

ABDOMINAL PAIN

What is it?

The subjective feeling of pain and/or discomfort in the abdominal region

What are the important factors of the patient's history?

1. Intensity, duration, character, location, radiation, timing of the pain
2. Occurrence of pain in association with eating or change in position
3. History of trauma, melena, blood in stool, nausea, vomiting, or diarrhea
4. Urinary tract symptoms (e.g., dysuria, frequency)
5. Ob/gyn symptoms (e.g., vaginal discharge, pelvic pain)

What are the important factors of the physical exam?

Observation: Look for distension, retraction, discoloration, and protrusions.
Auscultation: Listen for presence or absence of bowel sounds as well as their intensity, pitch, location, and frequency; also listen for bruits.
Percussion: Percuss to determine organ size, amount of air in the gut, and presence of ascites.
Palpation: Palpate for tenderness (location, intensity, association with guarding and/or rebound), organ

	enlargement, prominent aortic pulsations (> 5 cm), and masses. Rectal and/or pelvic exams are frequently indicated.
What laboratory tests are usually indicated?	CBC with differential, electrolytes, renal function, LFTs, amylase, lipase, urinalysis, beta HCG
What other diagnostic tests are commonly used?	Abdominal series, which involves flat and upright (or decubitus) plane radiograph of the abdomen with a chest radiograph (CXR), is used. Ultrasound, contrast studies (e.g., UGI, barium enema), and CT are other radiologic studies frequently performed. Peritoneal lavage and laparoscopy are surgical techniques that may be useful in the diagnosis of abdominal pain.
What are the common causes?	
GI causes?	Infection (e.g., gastroenteritis, diverticulitis, appendicitis, peptic ulcer disease, gastroesophageal reflux, inflammatory bowel disease, irritable bowel syndrome, pancreatitis, gallbladder disease, volvulus, cancer
Genitourinary causes?	Cystitis, pyelonephritis, calculi of the renal system, pelvic inflammatory disease, ovarian cyst, ovulation pain, ectopic pregnancy, cancer
Vascular causes?	Ischemic bowel disease, dissecting aortic aneurysm, MI, pulmonary embolism (PE)
Pulmonary causes?	Pleurisy, pneumonia
Psychiatric causes?	Anxiety, depression, personality disorder, drug abuse, Munchausen syndrome
Neurologic causes?	Autonomic dysfunction, motility disorders, herpes zoster, nerve root compression syndromes
Metabolic/toxic causes?	Lead toxicity and porphyria
What are the admission criteria?	Reasonable suspicion of a problem that would require urgent or emergent

surgical intervention; any acute condition requiring IV fluids, medications, antibiotics and/or blood products; moderate-to-severe pain of unknown etiology, particularly in a patient with a social situation that makes quick follow-up difficult (e.g., lack of transportation, excessive distance from the hospital); hemodynamic instability; mental status changes; evidence of acute blood loss; suspected MI or PE; moderate pain of unclear etiology

Helpful hints

In up to 80% of cases, history provides an accurate diagnosis. Avoid administering sedative analgesics until diagnosis is determined; they may alter the exam, the patient's ability to perceive changes in his symptoms, or both. Frequently repeat exam (every 30–60 minutes) and carefully document findings, especially for individuals with acute abdominal pain. Obtain surgery consult early in course of illness if disease requiring surgical treatment is suspected.

CHEST PAIN

What is it?

Subjective feeling of pain, discomfort, tightness, or pressure in the chest region

What are the important factors of the patient's history?

1. Quality, location, and duration of the pain
2. PART MAT—Changes in symptoms with
   Position
   Activity
   Respiration
   Trunk movement
   Meals
   Ambient **T**emperature

What diagnostic tests are commonly used?

EKG, CXR, arterial blood gases (ABGs), echocardiogram, exercise stress test, cardiac isoenzymes, UGI, esophagogastroduodenoscopy (EGD), esophageal manometry/pH studies, and urine drug screen

What are the common causes?	
Cardiac?	Ischemia, pericarditis, MVP, aortic dissection
Esophageal?	Reflux, spasm, esophagitis, cancer
GI?	Gastritis, peptic ulcer disease (PUD), cancer
Pulmonary?	Pneumonia, pleurisy, pneumothorax, PE
Musculoskeletal?	Costochondritis, rib fracture, intercostal muscle strain, cervical/thoracic disk disease
Psychiatric?	Anxiety, depression, personality disorder, cocaine abuse
Dermatologic?	Herpes zoster
What are the admission criteria?	Suspected MI or PE, evidence of acute blood loss, significant pneumothorax, respiratory distress, mental status changes, signs or symptoms of hemodynamic instability

Helpful hints

1. Suspected MI is a historical diagnosis; the initial diagnostic tests can support this diagnosis but not conclusively rule out MI.
2. Early herpes zoster can cause pain before the lesions erupt.

DIZZINESS

What is it?	The subjective sensation of feeling lightheaded, unsteady, off balance, or spinning
What are the important factors of the patient's history?	1. Duration, frequency, and exact nature of symptoms (e.g., presence of vertigo) 2. Associated symptoms—hearing loss, tinnitus, palpitations, incoordination,

speech difficulty, numbness, weakness, chest pain, or symptoms associated with movement

3. Medication, particularly antihypertensives and aminoglycosides, can contribute to and/or precipitate dizziness.

What diagnostic tests are commonly used?

Orthostatic BP (lying, sitting, and standing), CBC, thyroid profile, EKG, echocardiogram, audiometry, tympanometry, CT/MRI, EEG

What are the common causes?

Vestibular?

Labyrinthitis, Meniere disease, benign positional vertigo, toxins (e.g., aminoglycosides)

Eighth-nerve disease?

Acoustic neuroma

Brain-stem disease?

CVA, tumor, demyelinating or degenerative disease

Cerebellar disease?

Partial complex seizures, normal pressure hydrocephalus

Cardiac?

Arrhythmias, ischemia, valvular disease, hypertension

Metabolic?

Thyroid disease, anemia, hypoglycemia

Psychiatric?

Depression, anxiety, somatization disorder

What are the admission criteria?

Evidence of serious or unstable cardiac or neurologic disease; significant functional impairment, particularly if etiology is unclear; dizziness progressing to syncope in middle-age or elderly patients

Helpful hints

Vestibular disease is the most common cause of dizziness, and psychiatric disorder is the second most common cause. Complaints of dizziness increase with age. Fifty percent of patients have multiple contributing factors. If vertigo is present, first focus on the vestibular system (inner ear).

DYSPNEA

What is it?	The subjective feeling of shortness of breath, having difficulty breathing, or both. It is often confused with rapid breathing (tachypnea).
What are the important factors of the patient's history?	1. Duration and frequency of the symptoms 2. Associated symptoms—chest pain, nausea, vomiting, diaphoresis, cough, wheezing, leg pain, abdominal pain, trauma 3. Other medical conditions, recent surgery, and/or medications
What are important physical findings?	Respiratory rate, BP, respiratory sounds (wheezing, stridor, retractions), skin color (cyanosis), lung sounds, heart sounds (murmurs), pulsus paridoxus, and jugular venous distention (JVD)
What diagnostic tests are commonly used?	CXR, ABGs, EKG, V/Q scan, CBC, peak flow, echocardiogram, and cardiac isoenzymes
What are the common causes?	
Pulmonary?	Infection, asthma, COPD, pneumothorax, PE, foreign body aspiration
Cardiac?	Ischemia, pericarditis
GI?	Profound blood loss, ruptured viscous, cholelithiasis
Immunologic?	Anaphylaxis
Psychiatric?	Anxiety/panic, paranoid states, hypochondriasis, stimulant abuse
What are the admission criteria?	1. Suspected MI or PE; worsening CHF 2. Bronchospasm in a patient who does not quickly respond to initial therapy or in a patient with questionable follow-up (e.g., noncompliant patient, patient without transportation) 3. Infant less than 2 months of age with fever

4. Profound hypoxia of any cause
5. Paranoid/anxious patient who is a danger to self or others
6. Any condition requiring IV therapy or surgical intervention
7. Hemodynamic instability

FATIGUE

What is it?	The subjective feeling of lack of energy, tiredness, weakness, and/or lethargy
What are the important factors of the patient's history?	1. Duration and frequency of the fatigue as well as mitigating factors 2. Associated symptoms—fever, weight change, dyspnea, chest pain, dizziness, syncope 3. Work and exercise habits 4. Other medical conditions 5. Detailed sleep history
What are important physical findings?	Thyromegaly, JVD, abnormal heart or lung sounds, abdominal organomegaly, lymphadenopathy, jaundice, edema, joint effusion, muscle tenderness, affect
What diagnostic tests are commonly used?	CBC, TSH, and others (e.g., CXR, echocardiogram, sleep study, antibody titers) pending careful history and physical exam
What are the common causes?	
Cardiac?	CHF, ischemia
Respiratory?	COPD, sleep apnea
Endocrine?	Hyper- and hypothyroid, diabetes mellitus
Lifestyle?	Poor physical conditioning
Infectious disease?	Endocarditis, hepatitis, HIV, mononucleosis, TB, Lyme disease
Hematologic?	Anemia, malignancy

Oncologic?	Any malignancy
Musculoskeletal?	Inflammatory arthritis, chronic fatigue syndrome
Psychiatric?	Depression, anxiety, somatization, substance abuse
Iatrogenic?	Medication
Helpful hints	Fatigue is rarely related to significant illness. Fifty percent of cases are secondary to psychiatric conditions. Minimal initial workup is best if no obvious underlying etiology is found following careful history and physical exam.

FEVER

What is it?	Elevation of core body temperature caused by a change in the *set point* in the hypothalamus—i.e., NOT hyperthermia, which is temperature elevation caused by an inability to dissipate heat effectively secondary to internal or environmental factors, such as heat stroke
What body temperature is considered elevated?	Rectal temperature 38 C (or 100.4 F)
What adjustments are made for oral and axillary readings?	Oral temperature + 0.6 C (or 1 F) = rectal temperature Axillary temperature + 1.1 C (or 2 F) = rectal temperature
Why does the set point change?	Pyrogens released from peripheral tissues stimulate prostaglandin-mediated pathways in the hypothalamus to change the set point.
What are the common causes?	Remember the mnemonic **MAIDS: M**alignancy, **A**utoimmune disease, **I**nfection, **D**rugs, **S**oft tissue injury/ inflammation (MAIDS)

What is the treatment?	It is essential to treat the underlying cause for true resolution of fever. Prostaglandin inhibitors, such as acetaminophen and NSAIDS (e.g., aspirin, ibuprofen) are effective.
What should you remember before treating a fever?	Fever is part of the immune response to infection; treatment *may* help infecting organisms survive longer and/or decrease antibody response. Treatment with aspirin is associated with Reye syndrome in children with certain infections, such as influenza and chickenpox. Fever induces tachycardia and increased myocardial oxygen demand; treatment may be beneficial to persons with underlying cardiac disease. Treatment frequently helps people feel better but doesn't shorten the illness.
What are significant complications to fever?	Brain injury can occur if rectal temperature > 41 C (or 106 F). Some children have febrile seizures.
What are the admission criteria?	Admission depends on underlying condition and its severity. Rarely admit anyone just for fever.

NAUSEA AND VOMITING

What is nausea?	The sensation that one is going to vomit
What is vomiting?	Gastric contents being forcefully expulsed through the mouth
What are the important factors of the patient's history?	1. Duration of symptoms (acute versus chronic) 2. Timing related to meals 3. Color and contents of vomit 4. Associated symptoms—chest and/or abdominal pain, fever, diarrhea, weight loss, previous surgery, headache, pregnancy 5. Other medical conditions
What are the causes of nausea and vomiting?	Nausea and vomiting can be responses to abnormalities in any organ system. A

careful history and physical exam usually direct further studies to the appropriate organ system. Medications are a particularly common cause of nausea.

What are the admission criteria?

Patients with nausea or vomiting associated with hemodynamic instability, acute blood loss, fluid/elecrolyte abnormalities and/or cardiac ischemia

What are potential complications of vomiting?

Dehydration, electrolyte and acid–base abnormalities, pulmonary aspiration, tear in the wall of the stomach (Mallory-Weiss tear)

What are the treatment options?

Identification and treatment of the underlying cause is the best therapy. Symptoms can be controlled with antiemetics [e.g., dopamine antagonists (promethazine, etc.) and anticholinergics (hydroxyzine, etc.)].

SYNCOPE

What is it?

A sudden, transient loss of consciousness

What are important factors of the patient's history?

1. Length of time unconscious
2. Presence of jerky movements or urinary or fecal incontinence
3. Associated symptoms—cough, micturition, chest pain, palpitations, anxiety
4. Exacerbation/occurrence of symptoms when patient changes position or posture or during exercise
5. Known history of cardiac disease (e.g., ischemia, rheumatic disease, valvular disease)
6. Medications, other medical conditions, family history of sudden death

What are important physical findings?

Orthostatic BP (lying, sitting, standing), bradycardia with carotid pressure, heart murmur

What diagnostic tests are commonly used?

EKG, echocardiogram, Holter monitor, EEG, urine drug screen, CT/MRI

What are the common causes of syncope?

Syncope is most commonly associated with excessive parasympathetic activity (vasodilatation/bradycardia)—vasovagal syncope, postural syncope, cough syncope, micturition syncope, and carotid sinus hypersensitivity. Neurologic causes include seizures. Cardiac causes include ischemia, heart failure, arrhythmias, asymmetric septal hypertrophy, and valvular disease.

What are the admission criteria for patients with syncope?

Evidence of cardiac ischemia or significant arrhythmia; elderly persons with new onset syncope of unclear etiology; significant injury secondary to loss of consciousness; any process that places the patient at significant risk, such as new onset seizures in an adult or unclear ability/willingness for appropriate follow-up

Helpful hints

Careful history taking is extremely important. Cerebrovascular disease rarely causes syncope. Syncope in elderly patients has worse prognosis. In addition, 25% of syncope cases are secondary to cardiac conditions. In 40% of syncope cases, no etiology is found. Many states have driving restrictions for individuals with syncope.

4

Common Cardiovascular Problems

ARRHYTHMIA

What is it?

An abnormality of the rate, rhythm, or conduction of electrical impulses in the heart

What are common signs and symptoms?

Palpitations (i.e., the sensation that the heart is beating "hard," fast, or doing "flip-flops" in the chest) are the most common complaint, although arrhythmias are often asymptomatic. The patient may also have chest pain, dyspnea, dizziness, and/or syncope. The pulse is usually fast (> 100 bpm) or slow (< 60 bpm), with or without irregularity; accelerated junctional rhythms or atrial tachycardias with block can have a normal pulse rate and rhythm. The blood pressure (BP) can be low, normal or high.

What may the heart and lung exam show?

Heart exam will correlate with the rate and rhythm of the pulse and may reveal murmurs, rubs, or abnormal heart sounds. Lung exam may reveal crackles, wheezes, and/or effusion. Jugular venous distention may be present. However, the exam may be completely normal.

What is the most common cardiac condition that can cause arrhythmias?

Ischemic heart disease

Other cardiac conditions that can cause arrhythmias?

Cardiac chamber enlargement
Valvular disease
Pericardial disease

CHF
Hypertension

What are common, non-cardiac causes of arrhythmias?

Electrolyte abnormalities, thyroid disease, CNS abnormalities, respiratory disease, drug abuse (particularly cocaine) and therapeutic drug side effects are other relatively common causes of arrhythmias.

What are common diagnostic tests?

The electrocardiogram (EKG) will identify the type of arrhythmia (if it is persistent) in most cases. A 24-hour Holter monitor or an event monitor may be needed to document a paroxysmal arrhythmia and clearly associate it with symptoms. Once the arrhythmia is identified, the etiology of the arrhythmia should be sought. Echocardiogram, serum electrolytes, thyroid-stimulating hormone (TSH), chest radiograph (CXR), urine drug screen, arterial blood gases (ABGs), and serum drug levels should be considered according to the symptoms and physical exam.

How can common arrhythmias be classified?

Classify arrhythmias into subgroups according to:
1. **Rate:** bradyarrhythmias (< 60 bpm) or tachyarrhythmias (> 100 bpm)
2. **Origin:** atrial, junctional, or ventricular

What are the three most common bradyarrhythmias, and what are their characteristics?

1. **Sinus bradycardia.** The rhythm originates in the sinus node, but the rate is < 60 bpm. This can be a normal variant (e.g., training effect in athletes), iatrogenic (e.g., related to drugs, such as β-blockers) or abnormal (e.g., sick sinus syndrome, hypothyroidism).
2. **Atrioventricular (AV), or junctional, rhythm.** This rhythm originates in the AV node, usually secondary to a disease process that impairs sinus node function. The periodicity of the AV node is less than 60 impulses per minute (40–60 bpm), resulting in bradycardia.

Accelerated junctional rhythm can be > 60 bpm.

3. **Idioventricular rhythm.** This rhythm originates in the ventricle secondary to disease in the sinus and AV nodes. The periodicity of this rhythm is 20–35 bpm. Patients with this rhythm are frequently symptomatic (lightheaded, dizzy, syncopal). Accelerated idioventricular rhythm can be > 60 bpm.

How are bradyarrhythmias treated?

Management involves identifying the underlying cause and treating it, if possible. Artificial pacemaker (external or internal) is used if correcting the underlying cause is not possible or if there is irreversible injury (e.g., ischemic injury).

What are four common tachyarrhythmias, and what are their characteristics?

1. **Sinus tachycardia** results from increased rate of firing of the sinus node, which is usually caused by external agents (e.g., sympathetic nervous system, fever, drugs, hyperthyroidism) affecting the sinus node.

2. **Supraventricular tachycardia (SVT).** Most narrow QRS complex tachyarrhythmias are grouped into this category. They usually result from re-entry phenomena in the atria or AV node. The re-entry pathways are usually secondary to ischemia or drugs (e.g., digoxin) in older patients. SVT can be associated with hypotension and hemodynamic compromise in these older patients, so prompt evaluation and treatment are indicated. Young patients with paroxysmal atrial tachycardia (PAT) usually have symptoms (e.g., palpitations, dizziness) but otherwise normal hearts.

3. **Atrial fibrillation.** This rhythm is secondary to a very rapid intrinsic atrial pacemaker (rate 400–600 bpm) with varying degrees of AV block, leading to an irregular rate. It can be

associated with cardiac conditions [e.g., ischemia, congestive heart failure (CHF), valvular disease] or noncardiac conditions (e.g., hyperthyroidism, alcohol effects).

4. **Ventricular tachycardia.** This rhythm results from re-entry phenomena in the ventricle. Because it is most frequently associated with active ischemia, it is frequently related to hypotension and can decompensate into even less stable rhythms (ventricular fibrillation). Ventricular tachycardia is a potentially life-threatening arrhythmia, even in an asymptomatic patient. Emergency evaluation, treatment, and intensive care monitoring are indicated.

What are general considerations in the treatment of tachyarrhythmias?

Treatment of tachyarrhythmias is best accomplished if the underlying cause is identified and treated. However, because SVT in older patients, atrial fibrillation, and ventricular tachycardia can be related to hemodynamic compromise, treatment often needs to be initiated before evaluation of etiology.

What medications are used to treat the common tachyarrhythmias?
SVT?

Pharmacologic therapy of SVT can include adenosine, esmolol, calcium channel blockers (especially verapamil) and digoxin (except with pre-excitation syndromes, such as Wolff-Parkinson-White syndrome).

Atrial fibrillation?

Pharmacologic therapy of atrial fibrillation involves acute rate control with IV verapamil, diltiazem, esmolol, or digoxin. Digoxin is the agent of choice for control of chronic atrial fibrillation.

Ventricular tachycardia?

Pharmacologic therapy of ventricular tachycardia can include lidocaine, bretylium, and procainamide.

What nonpharmacologic therapy is used to treat tachyarrhythmias?

SVT can respond to carotid massage or Valsalva maneuver. SVT, atrial fibrillation, and ventricular tachycardia can all be treated with electrical cardioversion, but this procedure is reserved for patients with hemodynamic compromise.

What are the admission criteria for a patient with arrhythmia?

All patients with hemodynamic compromise secondary to arrhythmias should be admitted. This may require intensive cardiac care in a coronary care unit (CCU) and usually requires continuous cardiac monitoring until patient and rhythm stabilize. Patients with new onset atrial fibrillation and any arrhythmia associated with symptoms of active ischemia should be admitted and evaluated for ischemia. Cardiology consult is helpful in these cases.

Helpful hints

Atrial fibrillation is associated with a high incidence of thromboembolic stroke in patients older than 65 years of age. These patients should be treated with chronic warfarin therapy (INR 2.0–3.0) if no contraindications exist.

CONGESTIVE HEART FAILURE (CHF)

What is it?

It is a clinical syndrome secondary to the inability of the heart to maintain an adequate cardiac output.

What are the hemodynamic abnormalities in CHF?

The clinical signs and symptoms result from increasing left ventricular pressures created by the inadequate cardiac output. This leads to pulmonary vascular congestion with transudate of fluid into the alveoli, followed by increased right heart pressure and peripheral venous pressure increases, resulting in hepatic congestion and peripheral edema.

What are important historical factors?

History of hypertension, coronary artery disease (CAD), arrhythmias, thyroid disease, alcohol and/or other substance abuse, discontinuation of medications, medications that impair myocardial contractility (β-blockers, calcium channel blockers, Adriamycin), excess salt in the diet, recent infection, rheumatic fever,

recent pregnancy, malignancy, and/or
history of autoimmune disease

**What are common signs
and symptoms?**

Symptoms
Dyspnea [including orthopnea (i.e.,
   dyspnea when lying down), paroxysmal
   nocturnal dyspnea (PND), and
   dyspnea with exertion]
Lower extremity edema and/or cough
   productive of watery or frothy sputum
Chest pain, palpitations, and syncope or
   near syncope can be associated with
   some of the causes of CHF.

Signs
Tachycardia
Jugular venous distention (JVD)
Presence of a third heart sound (S_3)
Bilateral crackles on lung exam
Pitting edema of the feet and/or legs
Elevated BP is often found, but the
   patient may also have normal or low
   BP.
Low oxygen saturation documented with
   percutaneous oximetry (with or
   without cyanosis)

**What are the two types of
CHF?**

1. Systolic dysfunction
2. Diastolic dysfunction

**What hemodynamic
abnormalities are
associated with each?**

1. **Systolic dysfunction,** as the name
   indicates, is the inability of the heart
   to generate sufficient systolic forces
   to maintain an adequate cardiac
   output. The myocardium is weakened
   and often damaged. The heart is
   dilated, shifting myocardial
   contractility to the downward slope of
   the Starling curve. The diminished
   contractile force leads to an increased
   residual volume that is reflected in a
   decreased ejection fraction (EF).
   Preload increases due to the
   increased pulmonary and right heart
   pressures associated with decreased
   EF. Afterload increases from
   compensatory mechanisms, mainly
   vasoconstriction, that attempt to
   maintain blood pressure despite
   decreasing cardiac output.

2. **Diastolic dysfunction** is caused by the inability of the myocardium to appropriately relax during diastole, which leads to decreased cardiac output secondary to inadequate stroke volume (SV) from poor ventricular filling. Left ventricular hypertrophy (LVH) is a common finding with diastolic dysfunction. EF is normal or increased.

What are the common causes of CHF?

Remember: CHF is a clinical syndrome. An etiology should always be sought and identified in patients with CHF.

Common causes of CHF include ischemia, hypertension (HTN), uncompensated hyper- or hypothyroidism, arrhythmias, alcohol, infections, valvular disease, and drugs (both drugs of abuse and therapeutic agents).

What are less common causes?

Less common causes are recent pregnancy, malignant infiltration, and autoimmune disease.

What are common diagnostic tests?

CXR, EKG, echocardiogram, 24-hour Holter monitor, cardiac catheterization, thyroid panel, blood alcohol, urine drug screen, and therapeutic drug levels should be considered, depending on the history and physical findings.

What will the CXR show?

An overall increase in vascular markings, especially in the upper lung fields (cephalization of flow). An interstitial infiltrate may be present and is usually bilateral. The infiltrate begins in the lower lung fields and progresses upward as the failure worsens. Wave-like horizontal lines, Kerley's-B lines, can be seen in the lung fields if the infiltrate is especially intense. Pleural effusions can be seen. Cardiomegaly is often present from either a dilated left ventricle (systolic dysfunction) or LVH (diastolic dysfunction).

Why is the EKG useful?

It can document arrhythmia, LVH, and/ or ischemia.

What is the role of the echocardiogram?

It is the noninvasive test of choice to document systolic versus diastolic dysfunction (EF), LVH, and valvular heart disease. Segmental wall motion abnormalities indicate ischemia. Atrial enlargement can indicate predisposition to atrial arrhythmias, such as atrial fibrillation.

How can the 24-hour Holter monitor be useful?

It can help document paroxysmal arrhythmias that precipitate CHF.

How is cardiac catheterization useful?

It is the gold standard for documenting ischemic disease, EF, and valvular heart disease (including pressure gradients across valves). Also, the cardiologist can perform myocardial biopsy if needed for etiology (e.g., in viral cardiomyopathy).

TREATMENT

How is CHF treated?

Treatment of the underlying etiology is the most effective long-term management strategy. Otherwise, therapy is directed by whether the CHF is secondary to systolic or diastolic dysfunction.

What are general principles for treating systolic dysfunction?

Preload and afterload reduction, with inotropic agents, if needed

What pharmacological agents are used for these principles?
    Preload reduction?

Loop diuretics, such as furosemide, are first-line agents for systolic dysfunction. Nitroglycerin (topical or oral) can also reduce preload but this is used as a second-line agent (although it may be very useful in patients with ischemia contributing to their CHF).

    Afterload reduction?

Angiotensin-converting enzyme (ACE) inhibitors reduce morbidity and mortality in patients with systolic dysfunction and should be used in all patients with CHF secondary to systolic dysfunction unless there is a strong contraindication, such as allergy to ACE inhibitors. Hydralazine is a second-line agent reserved for patients who cannot tolerate ACE inhibitors.

Inotropic agents?

Digoxin is the first-line inotrope and has proven benefit for patients with systolic dysfunction. It has a narrow therapeutic window, which dictates documenting serum levels and remaining aware of potential drug interactions. There are several inotropic agents in development at the present time, but trials documenting safety and efficacy have not been completed. Negative inotropic agents are contraindicated.

What are the general principles for treating diastolic dysfunction?

Diastolic dysfunction is treated with agents that decrease the chronotropic and inotropic forces of the myocardium. This gives more time for diastolic filling of the left ventricle and also permits better myocardial relaxation during diastole. Control of HTN is also important.

What pharmacologic agents are used for these principles?

Calcium channel blockers and β-blockers are the first-line agents. Diuretics, ACE inhibitors, and other agents are used for control of HTN as needed. Positive inotropic agents are contraindicated.

Helpful hints

1. Distinguishing between systolic and diastolic dysfunction is important, because therapy is different and agents used to treat one syndrome can negatively impact the other.
2. Patients with diastolic dysfunction and systolic dysfunction secondary to ischemia are at high risk for ischemic events. Aggressive risk-factor modification is indicated.

What are the admission criteria for a patient with CHF?

Hemodynamic compromise
Suspicion of active ischemia [e.g., evolving myocardial infarction (MI), unstable angina]
Uncontrolled or new arrhythmia
New onset of CHF with unclear etiology

Worsening symptoms despite appropriate therapy

Syncope

Thyroid storm and/or worsening symptoms in a patient with unclear or unreliable social support or transportation

CORONARY ARTERY DISEASE (CAD)

What is it?

CAD is any process that alters the ability of the coronary arteries to deliver adequate bloodflow (and, therefore, oxygen) to meet the metabolic demands of the myocardium. This is why it is also called ischemic heart disease.

What are the two functional divisions of CAD?

1. Large vessel (epicardial) disease
2. Small vessel (endocardial) disease

What is the significance of these two divisions?

Large vessel disease has multiple treatments (e.g., medication, angioplasty, surgery), whereas small vessel disease can usually only be treated with medication.

What are the risk factors for CAD?

There are five independent risk factors:
1. Family history of CAD
2. HTN
3. Smoking
4. Hypercholesterolemia
5. Diabetes mellitus

What other conditions are associated with CAD (but have not been shown to have definitive independent risk)?

Poor physical conditioning (lack of exercise)
Obesity
Increasing age
Stress

What are the causes of CAD?

Atherosclerosis (90%–95%)
Vasospasm (5%–10%)

What is atherosclerosis?

A process whereby lipids are deposited in the subintimal layer of an artery, leading to an inflammatory response with oxidation of the lipids by free radicals. A hard plaque results, which gradually enlarges and progressively occludes the lumen of the vessel.

How does atherosclerosis cause symptoms?

Initially, the plaque does not cause symptoms, because the lumen is not occluded enough to restrict bloodflow at rest or during periods of peak demand (e.g., vigorous exercise). However, as the plaque enlarges, it reaches a critical size at which it occludes the lumen to the degree that bloodflow is inadequate during periods of high demand. Therefore, the metabolic demand of the myocardium for oxygen is not met. When myocardial oxygen demands are not met, symptoms (usually chest pain) often occur. If the plaque enlarges enough, there will be symptoms at rest. Also, if platelets adhere to a large or ulcerated plaque or if there is vasospasm in a segment with plaque, the vessel can totally occlude. If total occlusion lasts longer than 20–30 minutes, MI (necrosis) occurs.

What are common signs and symptoms of cardiac ischemia?

Chest pain with or without radiation to the neck and/or left arm
Left arm or shoulder pain
Nausea
Dyspnea
Diaphoresis
(Association of any of these symptoms with activity or exercise increases the likelihood of CAD as does the association of nausea, dyspnea, and/or diaphoresis with "typical" chest pain.)

Describe the typical chest pain associated with CAD.

The pain is located in the substernal region and is described as a tight, squeezing, and/or pressure sensation. Patients often describe the feeling as if something or someone were sitting on their chest. The pain is associated with activity and/or exercise and relieved with rest.

What is another name for this type of chest pain?

Angina—it is the cardinal symptom of CAD.

What are three common clinical syndromes associated with CAD, and what are the characteristics of these syndromes?

1. **Stable angina** occurs at a stable frequency and duration and is responsive to anti-anginal agents. Duration of an episode is less than 20 minutes.
2. **Unstable angina** occurs in an increasing or unpredictable frequency and/or duration from a previously stable pattern. This type of angina is particularly worrisome, because it indicates worsening disease and can indicate impending MI. It is an urgent medical condition, requiring prompt evaluation and therapy.
3. **MI** is acute necrosis of myocardium. Common symptoms are crushing chest pain with nausea, diaphoresis, and/or radiation to the neck or left arm. Duration of symptoms is 20 minutes or greater. MI is a life-threatening medical emergency requiring immediate treatment.

What are common diagnostic tests for CAD?

EKG
Echocardiogram
Exercise stress test (EST) with or without radionuclide imaging or echocardiography
Serial serum cardiac isoenzyme levels
Cardiac catheterization

Do all patients with angina need cardiac catheterization?

No. Most will need an EST to determine the level of exercise that is safe for risk factor modification. However, cardiac catheterization may be reserved for patients with symptoms that are unresponsive to medical therapy, abnormal EST with radionuclide imaging or echocardiogram, or unstable angina and other clinical situations in which suspicion of critical stenoses with high risk of MI exists (e.g., a patient with recent MI).

TREATMENT

What are the general considerations in the treatment for CAD?	Therapy for CAD should be approached according to the applicable clinical syndrome—stable angina, unstable angina, or MI.
What is the goal of therapy for stable angina?	To decrease frequency of episodes of angina, prevent progression of disease to MI, and decrease mortality from MI if the patient's disease progresses

What pharmacologic agents are used to treat stable angina, and what are the benefits of each?

1. β-Blockers decrease frequency and duration of anginal episodes and decrease frequency of mortality from MI.
2. Aspirin decreases mortality from MI and decreases incidence of repeat MI. It does not change duration or frequency of angina episodes but should be used in all patients with increased risk factors for MI.
3. Nitrates. Short-acting nitrates used sublingually can abort anginal episodes and should be prescribed for all patients with angina. Topical and long-acting oral nitrates can decrease frequency of episodes. However, tolerance to the nitrate's effect develops with continuous usage and nitrate-free periods (e.g., overnight) should be included in the regimen.
4. Calcium channel blockers decrease the frequency of anginal episodes. However, they are usually contraindicated in acute MI; short-acting calcium channel blockers have had questions raised about their safety in patients with CAD and HTN. Careful consideration of these concerns should be used and discussed with patients when using these agents.

Describe risk-factor modification.

Carefully evaluate risk factors and modify those that have been shown to slow progression of CAD and/or decrease incidence of MI. Examples include smoking cessation, treatment of HTN, lipid modification, exercise program, and estrogen replacement therapy in postmenopausal women.

What are the general considerations for therapy of unstable angina?

Because it is often difficult to distinguish unstable angina from MI or impending MI, the patient should be monitored in CCU until symptoms resolve and acute MI has been ruled out. The patient should not be discharged until further evaluation of CAD with EST or cardiac catheterization has been scheduled.

What noninvasive agents are used to treat unstable angina, and what are the benefits of each?

1. Aspirin. Give promptly if patient is not already taking and has no contraindications.
2. Heparin prevents formation of thrombi that usually cause MI.
3. β-Blockers can be given orally or IV if patient has no contraindications and is not already taking one of these agents.
4. IV nitrates are effective.
5. Oxygen (increases oxygen available for ischemic myocardium)
6. Bed rest decreases total oxygen consumption, leaving more oxygen available for the myocardium.

What invasive methods are used to treat unstable angina?

Coronary angioplasty and coronary artery bypass are invasive treatments that attempt to open stenotic vessels or bypass stenotic lesions.

What are the general considerations for treating MI?

MI is a medical emergency, requiring emergent transportation and admission to CCU. Supportive therapy and recognition and treatment of complications are performed in the outpatient setting. Definitive therapy of EKG-confirmed MI with thrombolytics is usually reserved for the CCU, but initiation of thrombolytics in the outpatient setting is being investigated for situations in which transport time to the hospital is excessive.

How is an acute MI treated?

1. Aspirin. Have patient chew and swallow one 325-mg aspirin.
2. Oxygen at 4 L/min via nasal cannula
3. Bedrest
4. Morphine, 2–4 mg IV (or other parenteral analgesic). It treats pain and has an anxiolytic effect.
5. Thrombolytics. Lyse thrombi that obstruct the coronary artery and are thought to be the most common cause of acute MI. Thrombolytics decrease mortality by 50% if initiated < 3 hours after the onset of symptoms and by 10% up to 10 hours after onset of symptoms. So, initiate therapy ASAP after diagnosis.
6. Coronary angioplasty. Some centers report superior outcomes in patients who have angioplasty acutely to reopen the vessel causing the MI.
7. Lidocaine, bretylium, procainamide, and defibrillation treat arrhythmias that can occur as complications of MI.
8. Dopamine or dobutamine. Parenteral agent used to treat heart failure that can occur as a complication of MI.

What are the indications for use of thrombolytic therapy?

Acute EKG changes consistent with anterior or multifocal MI (i.e., a large MI). The benefit is less clear with inferior MI. There is no benefit in non-Q-wave MI or in patients with previous coronary artery bypass grafting.

What are the absolute contraindications of thrombolytic therapy?

Known bleeding diathesis
History of any type of cerebrovascular disease
Uncontrolled HTN (BP > 190/110)
Recent head or spine trauma or surgery
Pregnancy

What are the relative contraindications of thrombolytic therapy?

Recent major surgery
GI or GU bleeding
Diabetic retinopathy
Current warfarin therapy
Prolonged CPR
Age > 80, or > 70 if using t-PA

What are the admission criteria for a patient with CAD?	Any patient with unstable angina, MI, or suspected MI
Helpful hints	1. MI is a clinical syndrome. It can be confirmed by acute changes on EKG and/or elevated isoenzymes but not ruled out by a normal EKG or a normal initial isoenzyme level. Therefore, the decision to initiate monitoring and treatment is made on clinical grounds. 2. Thrombolytic therapy has a higher complication rate in elderly patients (especially CNS bleeding), but elderly patients also have a greater potential benefit due to higher mortality rate without treatment.

DEEP VENOUS THROMBOSIS (DVT)

What is it?	Formation of blood clots (thromboses) in the deep veins of an extremity; DVT most commonly refers to thromboses in the lower extremity
What are physiologic predisposing factors for DVT?	Virchow's triad: 1. Stasis 2. Hypercoagulability 3. Epithelial injury
What are common risk factors for DVT?	Remember the mnemonic **HAS BAIT:** **H**ypercoaguable states (e.g., malignancy) **A**utoimmune disease **S**urgery **B**edrest **A**nticardiolipin antibodies **I**mmobilization **T**rauma
What are common signs and symptoms of DVT?	Pain, tenderness, swelling, warmth of the involved extremity Palpable cord Homan's sign (i.e., calf pain with dorsiflexion of the foot)
What are the common diagnostic tests used?	1. Duplex Doppler ultrasound is the noninvasive test of choice.

2. Venogram: gold standard
3. Impedance plethysmography and radioisotope studies are less commonly used but can be helpful in some cases.

How is DVT treated?

IV heparin, IM low-molecular-weight heparin, oral warfarin, elevation of affected extremity, and warm compresses are used initially.

How is warfarin therapy managed?

Warfarin has a paradoxical effect on coagulation when initiated, so it must be given *with* heparin for 4–5 days, even if prothrombin time is therapeutic. Warfarin is continued for 4–6 months after the initial episode of DVT (longer if subsequent episodes occur). Outpatient therapy with low-molecular-weight heparin (IM injection bid) has been described recently and may be considered if the patient has adequate resources to ensure appropriate administration and follow-up.

What are common complications of DVT?

Pulmonary embolism (PE), chronic venous stasis, varicose veins

What are the admission criteria for a patient with DVT?

Any patient requiring treatment with IV heparin, including patients with documented clot above calf level or signs or symptoms of a clot above calf level awaiting diagnostic studies if they are poor candidates for low-molecular-weight heparin administered at home, should be admitted. This also includes patients who live a great distance from the hospital, do not have reliable transportation to the hospital, do not have a phone, or have a history of poor compliance with follow-up visits.

Helpful hints

1. Only thrombosis above calf level places patient at risk for embolization.
2. Anticoagulation therapy decreases incidence of clot propagation and PE; it does not cause the clot to dissipate.

HYPERTENSION (HTN)

What is it?	Sustained elevated BP: systolic > 140, diastolic > 90, or both
What is required for diagnosis?	Elevated measurement on three separate occasions over a 3-week period
What are common pitfalls to diagnosis?	Use of an inappropriate-size cuff for BP measurement Patient anxiety toward physician and/or office can artificially elevate BP ("white coat" HTN). Patient rushing to appointment can artificially elevate BP; allow patient to sit quietly for a few minutes before taking BP. (The latter two pitfalls can be overcome by intermittent measurements at home or by using a continuous BP monitor over several days.)
How many Americans have HTN?	50–60 million
What are the long-term complications of HTN?	MI, stroke, aortic dissection, peripheral vascular disease, renal failure, CHF
What are the short-term complications of HTN?	Usually none—however, if the BP is markedly elevated (systolic > 200, diastolic > 120), mental status changes, hemorrhagic stroke, and/or MI can occur acutely
What are the symptoms of HTN?	Usually none, which is why it is called "the silent killer" Occasionally headache, chest pain, epistaxis, neurologic symptoms (e.g., numbness, weakness), or nausea or vomiting occurs
What are the common signs of HTN?	S_4, loud aortic component of S_2, vascular changes of the retina
What are identifiable causes of HTN?	Renal disease, renal vascular disease, pregnancy, pheochromocytoma, and hyperaldosteronism

What percent of HTN occurs without identifiable cause?

95%—these patients are classified as having essential HTN; only patients with early onset of HTN, severe HTN, or HTN unresponsive to treatment should be evaluated for secondary causes; obesity, alcohol, tobacco, lack of physical conditioning can all contribute to elevated BP

What are common tests used in the initial evaluation of patients with HTN?

EKG, serum electrolytes, BUN, and creatinine to establish baseline values for future comparison and evaluate for evidence of end-organ damage (renal failure). In addition, cholesterol levels are useful for evaluating other risk factors for CAD. EKG is often obtained to establish a baseline for future comparison and evaluate for LVH.

TREATMENT

What are the two approaches to treatment for HTN?

Both nonpharmacologic and pharmacologic treatments are used. It is best to begin with nonpharmacologic treatment for patients with mildly elevated BP.

Is reduction of BP to normal levels the goal of treatment?

No. The goal of treatment is to prevent end-organ damage and reduce the incidence of MI, stroke, renal failure, and overall mortality. These goals are achieved by BP control.

What are nonpharmacologic treatments?

Exercise, weight reduction, reduced sodium intake, relaxation training, eliminating alcohol and tobacco use; a low-fat diet will not directly lower BP, but will help reduce weight and cholesterol

What classes of drugs are used to treat HTN?

Thiazide diuretics, β-adrenergic blockers (β-blockers), α-adrenergic blockers, ACE inhibitors, central sympatholytics, and calcium channel blockers all have shown to decrease BP effectively.

Which classes have been shown to actually reduce

Thiazide diuretics, β-blockers, and the central sympatholytic reserpine

**risk of MI and death?
Which class has been
implicated in increasing
mortality?**

Calcium channel blockers; however,
short-acting nifedipine was the only drug
studied. Other agents in this class have
different cardiovascular effects and may
not have similar negative effects.

**Why are thiazide diuretics,
β-blockers, and reserpine
not the only agents used?**

Despite being the cheapest agents and
the only agents with positive outcomes
data, their use is limited because of the
side effects (e.g., impotence, fatigue,
depression), metabolic effects (e.g.,
decreased potassium, increased glucose),
and negative effects on other diseases
(e.g., asthma, COPD, diabetes mellitus,
systolic dysfunction).

**Which agents should be
used first?**

It is still best to use thiazide diuretics, β-
blockers, and reserpine (in low doses) as
first-line agents unless a contraindication
exists. Switch to other agents as dictated
by side effects, and attempt to use
agents that help other conditions the
patient may have; for example, use an
ACE inhibitor in a patient with CHF, a
β-blocker in a patient with migraine
headaches, or an α-adrenergic blocker in
a patient with benign prostatic
hypertrophy.

**How does one choose a
second-line agent?**

It is best to use the cheapest agent that
will control the BP without side effects.
Also, as discussed, some agents may
benefit other diseases and be good
choices for patients with those problems.

**What are some of the
common side effects,
precautions, and
limitations of frequently
used antihypertensives?**
　Thiazide diuretics?

Fatigue, impotence, hypokalemia,
hyperglycemia, hyperlipidemia, and
hyperuricemia

　β-Blockers?

Fatigue, depression, promotes
bronchospasm in susceptible individuals,
hyperlipidemia; impairs metabolic
response to hypoglycemia and is
therefore dangerous in patients on
hypoglycemic agents, especially insulin;
contraindicated with other agents that

	impair AV conduction; less effective in African-Americans and elderly
ACE inhibitors?	Cough, hyperkalemia, angioedema; less effective in African-Americans (unless already on thiazide diuretic)
Calcium channel blockers?	No metabolic effects; questionable safety with short-acting nifedipine; verapamil and diltiazem impair AV conduction and should not be used with other agents with similar effect (e.g., β-blockers, digoxin).
Central-acting sympatholytics?	Fatigue, impotence, depression
α-**Adrenergic blockers?**	Fatigue, impotence, first-dose postural hypotension with some agents
What are the admission criteria for a patient with HTN?	Hypertensive crisis; admission is rarely indicated for HTN only
Helpful hints	1. Loop diuretics are not indicated for treatment of HTN. 2. Because HTN usually causes no symptoms, treatment should be tailored to avoid significant side effects, which improves patient compliance. 3. Hydrochlorothiazide (HCTZ) has a maximum antihypertensive effect at 25 mg; higher doses increase risk of hypokalemia but have little additional effect on BP.

HYPERTENSIVE CRISIS

What is it?	Marked elevation of BP that leads to acute impairment of end-organ function; also called malignant HTN
What BP level increases concern for hypertensive crisis?	Systolic > 200 and diastolic > 120

What symptoms indicate need for emergent intervention?

Mental status changes, chest pain or other symptoms of MI, visual disturbance, syncope

What physical findings indicate need for emergent intervention?

Papilledema, focal neurologic findings or other symptoms of stroke, new heart murmur, rales or other evidence of CHF

What diagnostic tests are used to evaluate patients with hypertensive crisis?

EKG, cardiac isoenzymes, renal function tests, electrolytes, echocardiogram, CXR, CT scan of head; test selection depends on presenting symptoms and their persistence despite therapy

What are general considerations in treating hypertensive crisis?

Urgency and aggressiveness of treatment depend on severity of symptoms. Most patients need a quiet environment, intensive nursing care, and continuous cardiac rhythm monitoring.

What medications are used to treat hypertensive crisis?

Oral—clonidine, captopril
IV—labetalol, nitroprusside infusion

What are the admission criteria for patients with hypertensive crisis?

All patients with malignant HTN should be admitted (usually initially to a CCU) until:
1. Adequate BP control has been established with oral medications
2. Enough time has passed to ensure rebound HTN does not occur
3. Significant, persistent end-organ damage (e.g., MI, CVA) has been adequately identified and/or treated

Helpful hints

1. Overly aggressive reduction of BP can lead to stroke, especially in older patients; therefore, avoid reducing the BP too low during initial therapy
2. Hypertensive crisis is defined by symptoms; patients with marked BP elevations but no symptoms can be treated with oral agents in the outpatient setting if they respond to therapy adequately.

PERIPHERAL VASCULAR DISEASE (PVD)

What is it?	Changes in the peripheral arterial vessels that lead to impairment in blood flow to peripheral tissues and, therefore, impaired oxygen delivery
What is the most common cause?	Atherosclerosis
Other causes?	Diabetes mellitus Poorly controlled, long-standing HTN Arterial smooth muscle proliferation or hyperreactivity Inflammation from autoimmune processes or infection
What are common risk factors for PVD?	Smoking Hypercholesterolemia HTN Diabetes mellitus Personal history of CAD and/or cerebrovascular disease Family history of vascular disease and/or autoimmune disease
What is the cardinal symptom of atherosclerotic PVD?	Claudication
What are other common signs and symptoms of PVD?	Skin ulcers of the lower extremities Abdominal pain with pulsating mass Diminished, absent, or asymmetric peripheral pulses Cool skin Bruits over vessels Difficult to control HTN and/or blanching of fingers with cold exposure
What is claudication?	Pain in the calf of the lower extremity that occurs with walking (i.e., angina of the leg) and that resolves with rest. It is caused by inadequate blood flow (i.e., inadequate oxygen delivery) to meet metabolic demands during exercise or activity. Anaerobic metabolism leads to

lactic acid accumulation and cramping pain.

What diagnostic tests are used in patients with suspected PVD?

1. Doppler ultrasound is the noninvasive test most frequently used, especially with the central vessels.
2. CT scan is often used to image the aorta, especially if aneurysm is suspected.
3. Comparing BP in the brachial artery and popliteal artery can confirm impaired flow; usually the BP in the popliteal artery is greater than the brachial artery.
4. Patients considering surgery will need angiography to confirm the location and extent of disease.
5. ESR and other lab tests for autoimmune processes (rheumatoid factor, antinuclear antibody) are used in appropriate situations.
6. Provocative testing is used for suspected Raynaud's vasospasm by placing the patient's hands in cold water and observing for blanching of the fingers.

What are common clinical syndromes of PVD?

Lower extremity PVD, aortic aneurysm, renal artery stenosis, Raynaud phenomenon, temporal arteritis

What are the etiology and common complications of each of these syndromes?
   Lower extremity PVD?

It is secondary to atherosclerosis and begins with claudication. It can progress to absent pulses, cool skin, ulcers of the foot and/or toes that don't heal, resulting in soft tissue infection, osteomyelitis, and gangrene. Amputations are common when disease progresses to this point.

Aortic aneurysm?

Long-standing, poorly controlled HTN can lead to distention of the aorta. When the diameter reaches a critical point (usually 5–6 cm), the risk of rupture greatly increases. Surgical treatment of abdominal aneurysms usually involves synthetic graft replacement. Treatment of thoracic aneurysms is difficult and controversial; surgical mortality is high, but attempts to repair after rupture are difficult.

Renal artery stenosis?

It can result from atherosclerotic plaque or arterial smooth muscle proliferation; proliferative disease can be bilateral. Hypoperfusion of the kidney and activation of the renin-angiotensin system lead to HTN that is severe for age and difficult to treat.

Raynaud phenomenon?

This is arterial smooth muscle hyperactivity in response to external stimuli. It is most commonly found in the vessels of the fingers, causing the skin of the fingers to blanch or turn blue when exposed to the stimulus (usually cold temperatures).

Temporal arteritis?

Autoimmune response leads to vasculitis in the temporal artery. Pain and tenderness in the artery is usually present, and the artery is often more prominent. Untreated, it can cause occlusion of the artery, resulting in blindness in the eye on the affected side. ESR is very high (60–100 mm/hr). Diagnosis is made with temporal artery biopsy. Treatment is initiated with high-dose prednisone ASAP with high clinical suspicion and/or ESR with biopsy arranged later to confirm diagnosis. (**Caution:** Inflammation can be focal and leave large portions of the artery unaffected. So, biopsy may give a false-negative result).

What are the medical treatments used for PVD?

Pentoxiphylline and aspirin are used with atherosclerotic disease. Risk-factor modification, especially smoking cessation and BP control, is important. Nifedipine is used for vasospasm. High-dose prednisone (60–80 mg/day) is used for vasculitis.

What are the surgical treatments?

Angioplasty, for both atherosclerotic and muscular hypertrophy lesions
Bypass with venous or synthetic graft

Helpful hints

1. Atherosclerotic PVD is the result of a systemic process. Patients must be considered at high risk for other manifestations of atherosclerosis, such as CAD and/or cerebrovascular disease. To establish surgical risk, appropriate evaluation for these associated conditions is important before surgery.
2. Without risk-factor modification (e.g., smoking cessation, HTN and lipid control), surgery for atherosclerotic PVD is almost useless due to high rates of recurrence.
3. Comparisons of upper and lower extremity BP can be done formally in a noninvasive vascular lab or in the office using a hand-held Doppler and a sphygmomanometer (BP cuff).

PULMONARY EMBOLISM (PE)

What is it?

Peripheral tissue that enters and moves through the venous system, through the right heart, and then lodges in a pulmonary artery

Where do emboli originate?

About 90% of PEs are from blood clots in the lower extremity (DVT). Other sources include fat and/or bone marrow from bone fractures, cannula and other foreign bodies from intravenous catheters, bits of tumor that erode into veins, air from IV accidents, pulmonary injury, and/or rapid ascent from SCUBA diving.

What are common signs and symptoms?

Dyspnea and pleuritic chest pain are the most common symptoms. Tachypnea, tachycardia, hemoptysis, fever, and diaphoresis are common physical findings.

What tests are used to diagnose PE?

EKG, ABGs, CXR, ventilation/perfusion nuclear (V/Q) scan, pulmonary angiography; tests looking for hypercoagulable states (e.g., prothrombin time, partial thromboplastin time, bleeding time, proteins S and C) are obtained in patients with recurrent PE.

What can the EKG show?

It is usually normal but may show evidence of right heart strain (e.g., S wave in lead I with Q wave with inverted T wave in lead III).

What will the ABGs show, and how should the results be evaluated?

Elevation of pH with low P_{CO_2} and low P_{O_2} (hypoxia with respiratory alkalosis; attempting to use specific cutoff values for pH and P_{CO_2} can be misleading, and it is best to interpret these values in light of the patient's clinical syndrome; an elevated $P(A - a)_{O_2}$ (i.e., alveolar to arterial oxygen gradient) is more sensitive than using a specific P_{O_2} value.

How does one calculate the $P(A - a)_{O_2}$ gradient?

The arterial P_{O_2} (Pa_{O_2}) is the P_{O_2} from the ABGs. The alveolar P_{O_2} (PA_{O_2}) is calculated from the following formula:

$$PA_{O_2} = PI_{O_2} - 1.25\, Pa_{CO_2}$$

where PI_{O_2} = the inspiratory partial pressure of oxygen, which is .21 at sea level, and Pa_{CO_2} = the CO_2 value measured in the ABG. Therefore, the A − a gradient = $PA_{O_2} - Pa_{O_2}$

What are normal values for the A − a gradient?

6 mm Hg for persons < 30 years old, and 15 mm Hg for persons > 60 years old

What can the CXR show?

A wedge-shaped infiltrate in patients with pulmonary infarction; however, the CXR is normal in most cases of PE

What will the ventilation/ perfusion (V/Q) scan show?

Because PE affects pulmonary vasculature, the V/Q scan will show deficits of perfusion in multiple areas or perfusion deficits in areas of normal ventilation. Preexisting lung disease and large PEs that cause atelectasis are the most common of many factors that can make interpretation of the V/Q scan difficult.

What will the pulmonary angiogram show?

It will show abrupt cutoff of flow in the affected artery. This is the gold standard of tests for PE; but because it is an invasive test, it carries significant morbidity and is reserved for situations where other tests are negative or inconclusive but the suspicion of PE is high.

How is PE treated?

IV heparin, supplemental oxygen, thrombolytics, warfarin

Helpful hints

1. Thrombolytics are usually reserved for patients with large PEs or significant hemodynamic compromise.
2. PIOPED study (*JAMA* 263: 2753–2759, 1990) outlines how V/Q scan and clinical suspicion of PE are used to decide if pulmonary arteriogram is needed.
3. Tumors more commonly cause hypercoagulability, leading to DVT and PE than actually being embolic material.

5   Common Ear Problems

CERUMEN IMPACTION

What is it?

Hard or soft waxy debris lodged in the external auditory canal (EAC)

What are the risk factors?

Family history of excess cerumen and/or impaction
Use of foreign bodies, such as cotton-tip swabs, to clean the EAC

What are the signs and symptoms?

Ear pain, decreased hearing

What diagnostic test is used?

Otoscopy

How is it treated?

Remove the cerumen by:
Irrigating with tepid water
Removing it manually with an ear curette
Administering a commercially prepared or homemade ceruminolytic; a weak solution of baking soda in water (e.g., 1 tsp of baking soda in 4 oz of water) is an excellent and inexpensive ceruminolytic.

What are the complications?

Otitis externa; hearing loss; perforation of the tympanic membrane (TM), which can occur when removing the impaction

How can it be prevented?

1. Some patients are wax producers. These patients should use a hygiene program of monthly cerumenolytics.
2. Discourage patients from using cotton-tipped swabs to clean the EAC.

HEARING LOSS

What is it?	The impairment or loss of the ability to hear sound in the normal range of intensity and frequency. Practically, it is based on the degree of social impairment (i.e., impaired ability to hear normal conversational speech), which can be correlated with audiometry findings.
What is slight impairment?	The person has difficulty hearing long-distance speech (e.g., at social occasions, at the theater). It represents a 10–30 decibel (dB) loss.
What is moderate impairment?	The person has some difficulty with short-distance speech and conversation. It represents up to a 60 dB loss.
What is severe impairment?	The person has no understanding of the conversational voice, but understands the amplified voice. It represents more than a 60 dB loss.
What is profound (total) impairment?	The person is an unable to hear and understand the spoken voice despite maximum amplification. It represents more than a 90 dB loss.
What are the two categories of hearing loss?	1. Conductive hearing loss—caused by occlusion of the EAC or diseases of the TM or middle ear, impairing conduction of sound to the sensory apparatus 2. Sensorineural hearing loss—caused by disease in the cochlea, CN VIII, auditory pathways, or auditory cortex
What are predisposing or risk factors?	Family history, noise exposure, ototoxic agent (e.g., aminoglycosides, aspirin, chemotherapeutics) exposure, age
What are the signs and symptoms?	Decreased ability to hear, tinnitus, cerumen in EAC, scarring of TM or decreased TM mobility on otoscopy

DIAGNOSTIC TESTS

What is an audiogram?

It is the gold standard test used to identify both frequency (pitch) and intensity (loudness;dB) deficits.

What are tuning fork tests?

Using a 512-Hz tuning fork, these tests identify unilateral versus bilateral hearing loss and otosclerosis versus sensorineural hearing loss.

How does the Weber test work?

The tuning fork is struck and placed on the vertex of the skull or elsewhere in the midline. When hearing is equal on both sides, the midline tuning fork sound is heard by a patient in the midline. This means that if hearing loss is present, it is bilateral. When hearing is unequal, the sound lateralizes to one side.

How does the Weber test sound lateralize with a sensorineural hearing loss?

The sound lateralizes to the normal ear, because of the impairment in the sensorineural pathway, which is not altered regardless of origin or conduction of sound.

With a conductive hearing loss?

The Weber test sound lateralizes to the impaired ear with a conductive hearing loss, because the ambient noise in the room "competes" with the bone-conducted sound from the tuning fork through the skull in the "good" ear. In the impaired ear, there is no competition because the normal conductive pathway is impaired and does not allow ambient noise to transmit to the cochlea. Because all of the sound from the tuning fork is conducted through the skull bones (bypassing the normal conductive apparatus in the middle ear), sensorineural pathways in both ears receive identical input from the tuning fork. Therefore, because the good ear also receives the ambient sound input that masks the sound from the tuning fork, the sound is louder in the impaired ear.

What does the Rinne test distinguish?	This test distinguishes conductive from sensorineural hearing loss for each ear.
How is the Rinne test administered?	The test involves lightly striking a tuning fork and placing the handle on the patient's mastoid process (bone conduction). When the sound becomes inaudible to a patient, the tuning fork is moved off the process and the prongs are held near the external ear (air conduction). A normal ear hears sound via air conduction louder and longer than via bone.
How do Rinne test results differ between patients with sensorineural hearing loss and those with conductive loss?	Sensorineural hearing loss has equally impaired air and bone conducted sound and, therefore, sound via air conduction remains louder and longer than via bone conduction as in a patient without hearing loss. Patients with unilateral sensorineural hearing loss have normal results on a Rinne test, even in the impaired ear. Conductive hearing loss interferes with air conduction of sound through the middle ear leaving neural pathways intact, which allows bone conduction via the skull to be louder. Therefore, sound heard via bone conduction is louder and longer than that heard by air conduction in an ear with conductive hearing loss.

TREATMENT

What is the treatment for lesions of the external ear canal?	If the EAC is blocked, remove cerumen or foreign body.
What is treatment for lesions of the middle ear?	1. Effusion with or without infection (otitis media) is the most common middle ear problem that can impair hearing. The effusion impairs conduction of sound through the middle ear and is usually treated with antibiotics and/or decongestants; however, tympanostomy with or without placement of tubes may be

needed for persistent effusion unresponsive to medical therapy.
2. Otosclerosis is fusion of the ossicles by proliferation of bone at their joints, which impairs the conduction of sound from the TM to the inner ear, leading to a conductive hearing loss. It is treated surgically by debriding the sclerotic bone, which restores the ability of the ossicles to transmit sound from the TM through the middle ear to the cochlea.
3. A cholesteatoma is the proliferation of epithelial tissue in the middle ear and requires surgery to débride the abnormal tissue. Hearing can be restored if the abnormal tissue is removed before destruction of vital structures (e.g., the ossicles, TM) occurs.

What is treatment for lesions of the inner ear?

Drugs, CNS infection, age (presbycusis), repetitive loud noise, etc. can lead to sensorineural hearing loss. These insults are usually not reversible and are treated with amplification (hearing aids). One exception to this is the acoustic neuroma which can be surgically removed leading to the possible restoration of normal or near normal hearing if removed before it causes permanent damage to CN VIII.

Helpful hints

1. Encourage patients to use ear protection when using loud equipment (e.g., a lawn mower) and to listen to the radio or recorded music (e.g., tapes, CDs) at a lower volume, especially with portable devices with earphones.
2. Avoid exposing patients to ototoxic drugs.
3. Periodically evaluate elderly patients for hearing loss (presbycusis; "old ears").
4. Otosclerosis often runs in families; ask about family history of hearing loss

OTITIS EXTERNA

What is it?	Inflammation of the EAC
What are three types?	1. Acute otitis externa, which is the most common and is usually bacterial 2. Eczematous otitis externa 3. Malignant otitis externa (invasive bacterial infection of the EAC), which is most commonly seen in patients with diabetes mellitus or in other immune compromised states
What are risk factors?	Hot/humid weather, use of a hearing aid, trauma, swimming (especially in lakes or rivers)
What are signs and symptoms?	Itching, sensation that the ear is occluded, otalgia, periauricular adenitis, purulent discharge, eczema of pinna
How is it diagnosed?	Otoscopy reveals erythema, inflammation, and edema, often with exudate. Movement of the pinna or pressure on the tragus causes significant pain.
What is the treatment?	**Acute otitis externa.** Topical antibiotic/steroid combinations are usually effective. Oral antibiotics are sometimes necessary if the infection is severe or topical antibiotics fail. **Eczematous otitis externa** responds to topical steroids. **Malignant otitis externa** requires parenteral antibiotics. *Pseudomonas* is a common pathogen and must be considered when choosing antibiotic coverage. It usually requires hospital admission. Otolaryngology consult may be helpful.
What are the complications?	TM perforation, cellulitis, sepsis
How can it be prevented?	Avoiding prolonged exposure to moisture (e.g., removing hearing aids at night, using alcohol drops after swimming)

Eliminating self-inflicted trauma to the canal by not using cotton-tip swabs or other foreign bodies to clean the EAC

Helpful hint

When treating with topical agents, use a wick in the canal if the edema is severe enough to almost obliterate the lumen of the EAC.

OTITIS MEDIA

What is it?

Inflammation of the middle ear; often caused by infection and usually associated with effusion

What are risk factors?

Being in day care
Formula feeding
Smoking in household
Family history of middle ear disease
Use of a pacifier

What are the signs and symptoms?

Ear pain, fever, decreased hearing, decreased TM motility, red and/or bulging TM

What diagnostic tests are used?

Otoscopy, which reveals red, bulging TM with effusion in the middle ear ("bulging" implies the loss of visualization of the bony landmarks on the TM)
Pneumatic otoscopy and/or **tympanometry** show decreased mobility of the TM due to effusion.

What are common pathogens?

Pneumococcus, *Haemophilus influenzae, Moraxella catarrhalis,* group A strep, *Staphylococcus aureus*

What are first- and second-line treatment options?

First-line agents: amoxicillin, trimethoprim/sulfamethoxazole
Second-line agents for resistant infections: amoxicillin plus clavulanic acid; cefixime; azithromycin

How is recurrent otitis media treated?

Three or more infections in 6 months may require daily prophylactic antibiotics for several months. Refer for surgery if

> 6 months bilateral otitis media with effusion or hearing loss > 25 dB. Surgery usually includes tympanostomy tubes and adenoidectomy.

What are complications?   TM perforation, mastoiditis, cholesteatoma, bacteremia

How can it be prevented?   Encourage parents to smoke outside or stop smoking.

Common Eye Problems

RED EYE

What is it?	The most common symptom of patients who present to primary care physicians with eye problems
What are common causes?	Many common eye problems, including infection (e.g., conjunctivitis), traumatic injury, acute glaucoma, corneal foreign body, and allergy and/or inflammation of structures of the eyelid cause swelling and/or inflammation of structures in or around the eye, making it appear red.
What are common symptoms?	Pain, change in visual acuity, diplopia, photophobia, and scotoma are all clinically important symptoms in a patient with a red eye.
What is involved in the evaluation of a red eye?	A careful examination is imperative to the evaluation of an acutely red eye. It should include examination of all structures: the lids (including eversion to examine the inner surface), conjunctiva, cornea, pupil, anterior chamber, vitreous, and retina.
What are some possible findings on examination of a red eye?	Conjunctival injection Refractive error Visual field defects Ocular movement and alignment Swelling of any structure in or around the eye Pupillary size, shape, or reactivity Corneal or anterior chamber discoloration or cloudiness Conjunctival, vitreous, or retinal hemorrhage

What common diagnostic tests are used?	1. Visual acuity testing with the Snellen eye chart 2. Fluorescein staining 3. Intraocular pressure measurement 4. Radiograph of the orbit (especially if metallic foreign body is suspected)
Why is visual acuity testing important?	Changes in visual acuity may be an important indicator of ocular abnormality, especially if the change is in the affected eye. It is important to question the patient about preexisting refractive error and use of corrective lens to understand the results of acuity testing.
What is fluorescein staining?	Fluorescein is an epithelial stain that fluoresces when exposed to cobalt blue light. It is placed in the eye, and then the cornea is examined under magnification with a cobalt blue light. Areas of abrasion fluoresce brightly from the accumulated stain.
How is intraocular pressure measured?	The cornea is anesthetized with a topical agent and a tonometer is used. The Schiøtz tonometer provides an indirect measurement of intraocular pressure, which is then translated into an intraocular pressure reading. This method of measuring intraocular pressure is operator-dependent and not as reliable as the direct method used by an ophthalmologist. If abnormal intraocular pressure is suspected clinically, it is best to refer the patient for a direct measurement.
What does elevated intraocular pressure indicate?	Glaucoma
What does low intraocular pressure indicate?	It may indicate penetrating injury with disruption of the cornea.
What is the treatment of a red eye?	Treat the underlying condition causing the red eye. If an etiology is not clearly identified, refer the patient to an ophthalmologist.

Helpful hints

1. Always document visual acuity before proceeding with other interventions, examinations, or evaluations. It is the only way to document that your exam, testing, and/or interventions did not cause worsening of the condition.
2. Do not use a mydriatic solution to dilate the pupil until you are certain that the patient does not have glaucoma, because this solution can precipitate acute glaucoma.
3. Do not use an agent that will affect the pupillary size or reactivity in any patient with head trauma, because these parameters are important in the ongoing evaluation of persons with head injury.

CONJUNCTIVITIS

What is it?

Inflammation of the bulbar and/or palpebral conjunctiva

What are three common causes?

1. Infection—bacterial or viral
2. Irritation—chemical or UV light
3. Allergy

What are common signs and symptoms?

Itching, redness, discharge, lid swelling, mild pain

Photophobia is not present, and visual acuity is usually unchanged.

The conjunctiva is usually infected and red, and the pupil is normal.

Preauricular adenopathy may be present with viral disease.

What diagnostic tests are used?

Gram stain and/or culture of the discharge

What treatment is used for viral conjunctivitis?

Isotonic saline drops can make the patient comfortable, but there is no specific treatment for viral disease. It is very contagious and strict hand washing is encouraged.

What treatment is used for bacterial conjunctivitis?

Topical antibiotic solution or ointment is used for 7–10 days. Otherwise, symptoms are treated as for viral disease.

What treatment is used for allergic conjunctivitis?

Systemic treatment for allergic rhinitis with antihistamines can help symptoms. Topical ophthalmic antihistamines and topical ketorolac may also help symptoms. Avoid using topical steroid preparations in the eye without supervision of an ophthalmologist.

What treatment is used for chemical conjunctivitis?

Chemical exposures are treated with immediate irrigation of the eye with copious amounts of water for 20–30 minutes, followed by prompt evaluation by an ophthalmologist. The offending agent should be identified and taken to the treating physician.

What treatment is used for conjunctivitis caused by excessive UV exposure?

Supportive care, including pain control and cycloplegia

Helpful hints

1. If the history is inconsistent with infection, the eye must be evaluated carefully for other possible etiologies of symptoms.
2. Photophobia with moderate-to-severe pain (especially in a patient with prolonged conjunctivitis symptoms) indicates possible iritis and requires referral.
3. Topical steroids are avoided, because herpetic conjunctivitis may be greatly exacerbated by steroids (local immune suppression) and lead to permanent corneal scarring. Corneal dendrites from herpetic infection are reliably seen only with slit-lamp exam, which usually requires ophthalmologic referral.

CORNEAL ABRASIONS AND FOREIGN BODIES

What is a corneal abrasion?

It is a superficial injury of the cornea that scrapes off the superficial layer of corneal epithelial cells.

What is a corneal foreign body?

It is a small piece of material (usually wood or metal) that imbeds into the superficial layers of the cornea. By definition, it does not completely penetrate the cornea.

What are common causes of a corneal abrasion?

Corneal abrasion is usually secondary to minor trauma. A glancing blow from a ball or other object and accidental injury from a finger into the eye during a sporting event commonly cause abrasions to the surface of the cornea.

What are common causes of a corneal foreign body?

Corneal foreign bodies are usually low-velocity projectiles that embed in the cornea. Chopping wood and hammering or grinding metal are examples of common activities that cause corneal foreign bodies.

How are these injuries prevented?

Use of appropriate eye protection (e.g., goggles, glasses, face shields) can prevent the majority of superficial corneal injuries.

What are common signs and symptoms?

Pain, foreign body sensation, erythema, and watery discharge; there is seldom significant swelling, and visual acuity, pupil shape, and reactivity are normal

What diagnostic tests are used?

Fluorescein staining is the test of choice and will identify most significant abrasions and foreign bodies. If a small, metallic foreign body is suspected, radiograph of the eye can help identify the location.

How are corneal abrasions treated?

Long-acting cycloplegics with topical antibiotics is the best treatment. Patches do not aid in healing and increase pain, so they should be avoided. Re-examination in 24 hours is also indicated.

How are corneal foreign bodies treated?

After the cornea is anesthestized with a topical agent, the foreign body is carefully teased out of the cornea using a fine-gauge hypodermic needle. After the foreign body is removed, the patient is treated for the remaining abrasion as described above.

Helpful hints	1. If you are concerned that a foreign body has penetrated the entire thickness of the cornea, do not remove it. Refer to an ophthalmologist.
	2. Small, high-velocity metallic foreign bodies can penetrate the globe. Heat associated with their separation from the host material can seal their entrance wound. High index of suspicion must be used if a corneal injury is associated with a high-velocity injury (i.e., metal on metal hammering). Radiograph of the globe will identify these metallic foreign bodies.
	3. Extensive or deep abrasions can cause scarring and should be referred.

HYPHEMA

What is it?	Hemorrhage into the anterior chamber of the eye
What causes it?	Blunt trauma to the eye
What are signs and symptoms of hyphema?	There is usually a recent history of trauma accompanied by pain, foreign body sensation, tearing, and/or photophobia.
What diagnostic tests are used?	Physical exam is the best test. The patient is placed in an upright, sitting position for several minutes, and the anterior chamber is examined for blood layering at the lower edge of the cornea. If the symptoms include evidence of corneal abrasion, fluorescein staining is indicated.
Why is the patient placed in a sitting position for the physical exam?	If the patient is lying down during the exam, the blood may distribute throughout the posterior portion of the anterior chamber and not be seen.
What is the main complication of hyphema?	Recurrent bleeding can lead to glaucoma and/or blood staining of the cornea.

How is hyphema treated?	The patient is placed at bed rest until the blood clears, because bed rest is thought to prevent further trauma and leakage of blood. Close follow-up with an ophthalmologist is important to evaluate and follow intraocular pressure. Severe or recurrent bleeding may require evacuation of the hematoma.
What kinds of drugs are contraindicated in a patient with hyphema?	Aspirin and other drugs that inhibit platelet aggregation or interfere with clotting

CHALAZION

What is it?	Chronic enlargement of a meibomian gland in the eyelid
What causes it?	Obstruction of the duct, usually due to inflammation
What are common signs and symptoms?	There may by pain and irritation initially, but most patients present for evaluation of a painless lump in the eyelid. If the chalazion is in the central/upper lid, some patients will have more chronic pain caused by irritation as the chalazion passes back and forth over the cornea when the eyelid is opened and closed. Examination shows a firm nodule in the eyelid, with easily moveable overlying skin.
How is a chalazion treated?	Initially, warm compresses are used to attempt to open the duct and allow return to normal function. If this is not successful, an ophthalmologist may need to inject the chalazion with steroids or incise and drain it.

HORDEOLUM (STYE)

What is it?	Acute infection of one or more of the glands of Zeis or Moll on the outer edge of the eyelid or of the meibomian glands on the internal portion of the eyelid

What distinguishes it from a chalazion?

The acute, suppurative course of an internal hordeolum (involving the meibomian glands) distinguishes it from a chalazion.

What causes it?

Acute glandular duct obstruction, often secondary to blepharitis

What is the most common causative organism?

Staphylococcus

What are common signs and symptoms?

Pain, redness, and swelling of the lid margin are the first symptoms. A small, localized area of induration and tenderness forms as the abscess matures. This area can drain purulent material. Pain decreases as the pus drains.

How is it treated?

Initially, warm compresses are used to help the involved area form a mature abscess. The abscess should then be incised and drained, and all contents should be removed. Systemic antibiotics may prevent abscess formation if started early enough. Topical antibiotics are not effective therapy.

GLAUCOMA

What is it?

A clinical syndrome characterized by increased intraocular pressure. It may lead to a wide spectrum of visual impairment, including blindness.

How is glaucoma classified?

Primary glaucoma is due to abnormalities in the eye that are congenital (e.g., as in infantile glaucoma), or it occurs secondary to an imbalance of the production and drainage of aqueous humor in the anterior chamber; the main problem is usually impaired drainage.

Secondary glaucoma occurs as a complication of other disease processes or injuries to the eye, such as uveitis, enlarged cataract, intraocular hemorrhage or tumor, trauma, central retinal vein occlusion, or prolonged use of intraocular steroids.

What are the three types of adult primary glaucoma?

1. Chronic open-angle glaucoma
2. Chronic angle-closure glaucoma
3. Acute angle-closure glaucoma

CHRONIC OPEN-ANGLE GLAUCOMA

What are important features of chronic open-angle glaucoma?

1. It is the most common type of glaucoma.
2. The eye appears structurally normal.
3. It almost always involves both eyes.

Describe the symptoms.

Symptoms are unreliable indicators of disease severity but may include halos around electric lights, mild headaches, impaired accommodation to darkness, and gradual loss of peripheral vision.

What are risk factors for chronic open-angle glaucoma?

It is more prevalent in persons older than 40 years of age, with severe myopia, with positive family history of glaucoma, with diabetes, or of African-American descent.

Why is screening needed in high-risk groups?

Because the patient may be asymptomatic until late in the course of the disease

What is the treatment?

Treatment usually is accomplished with eyedrops that decrease production of aqueous humor. Surgery is reserved for patients who don't respond to topical therapy.

ACUTE ANGLE-CLOSURE GLAUCOMA

What are important structural characteristics of this type of glaucoma?

Structural abnormalities are common: anterior chamber is usually shallow, the aqueous humor is turbid, the pupil is dilated and reacts poorly, and the cornea can be edematous. This type is often unilateral.

Describe the symptoms. Symptoms are prominent and include pain, vision impairment or loss, erythema of many structures (red eye), nausea, vomiting, and excessive lacrimation.

What may precipitate symptoms? Symptoms may be precipitated by agents that dilate the pupil. It obstructs the drainage system and acutely increases intraocular pressure.

What is the treatment? Treatment is initiated acutely with oral glycerin and/or carbonic anhydrase inhibitors to reduce and stabilize intraocular pressure. Oral carbonic anhydrase inhibitors are continued with topical miotics until surgery can be performed. Peripheral iridectomy or laser iridotomy are the procedures most often used and can be performed prophylactically in the uninvolved eye if the angle is narrow.

CHRONIC ANGLE-CLOSURE GLAUCOMA

What is it? Recurrent bouts of symptoms similar to acute angle-closure glaucoma but less severe

How is it treated? Acute management is the same as for acute angle-closure glaucoma, but topical agents are used until surgery is performed; chronic carbonic anhydrase inhibitors are contraindicated.

REFRACTIVE ERRORS

What is a refractive error? The inability of the eye to focus an external image clearly on the retina

What causes it? It can be secondary to anatomical problems of the eye (the globe is too narrow or too long) or due to inability of the lens to properly adjust the focus of the image in an eye that is anatomically normal.

What are common symptoms?

Blurred vision is the most common symptom. Difficulty with reading is also common.

What are the four most common refractive errors?

1. Hyperopia
2. Myopia
3. Astigmatism
4. Presbyopia

Define each of these four refractive errors.

1. **Hyperopia** (farsightedness) is difficulty with near vision in which the image is focused behind the retina. Hyperopia is due to a short eyeball or weak refractive ability of the lens.
2. **Myopia** (nearsightedness) is difficulty with distant vision in which the image is focused in front of the retina. It is due to an elongated eyeball or excessively strong refractive ability in the lens.
3. **Astigmatism** is unequal refraction in different meridians of the eye. Correction requires complex lenses that correct refraction differently along different axes.
4. **Presbyopia** is a hyperopia that occurs as a person ages. The lens loses it elasticity with time and, therefore, its ability to appropriately refract near images. Persons will hold reading material farther and farther away from the eyes in an attempt to overcome the change.

What diagnostic tests are used?

Vision testing (Snellen chart) for both near- and farsightedness is used to screen symptomatic patients. Ophthalmologists or optometrists have the ability to perform more detailed tests, and the patient should be referred if they fail screening.

How is it treated?

Corrective lenses are the most common treatment and can be mounted on frames (glasses) or placed on the cornea (contacts). Surgical treatment (radial keratotomy) can correct some refractive errors.

7 Common Endocrinologic Problems

DIABETES MELLITUS (DM)

What is it?

DM is a group of disorders in which the trademark is a propensity for hyperglycemia, secondary to an absolute deficit of insulin *or* to a relative deficit caused by "insulin resistance." They also share sequelae that may affect many organ systems and are thought to be associated with hyperglycemia.

What are the two most common types of DM?

Type I: insulin-dependent diabetes mellitus (IDDM)
Type II: Non-insulin-dependent diabetes mellitus (NIDDM)

Describe them.

Type I is an autoimmune disease that typically presents in the second decade. The patient develops an absolute insulin deficiency secondary to destruction of islet cells.
Type II is an adult-onset disorder in which patients develop hyperglycemia as a result of "insulin resistance"—i.e., the inability of their endogenous insulin to effectively store glucose.

What is a third, relatively common, type of DM?

Maturity-onset diabetes of the young (MODY), which typically presents in blacks who are 25–35 years of age and may include both an insulin-deficient state as well as an element of resistance. Secondary causes of DM include pancreatic disease, drug toxicity, and postsurgical diabetes.

80

Table 7-1. Comparison of Types I and II Diabetes Mellitus (DM)

Feature	Type I	Type II
Age of Onset	< 30 (usually 7–17)	> 40
Genetics	HLA-linked; 50% concordance in twins	Multifactorial; but twin concordance > 95%
Rate of Onset	Acute, commonly in DKA	Insidious, often presents after many years of unnoticed disease
Defect	Autoimmune destruction of insulin-producing cells	Insulin resistance
Epidemiology	Most prevalent in Caucasians and Scandinavians	Variable, but blacks > whites
Risk of DKA	High	Very low
Long-term DM complications	Common	Common

DKA = diabetic ketoacidosis; *IDDM* = insulin-dependent diabetes mellitus; *NIDDM* = non-insulin-dependent diabetes mellitus.

What lab test is most useful in differentiating type I from type II?	A C-peptide level measured before and after stimulation with glucagon can indicate the pancreas' capacity for insulin production.
What symptoms should alert the clinician to the possibility of DM?	Although DM can present in different ways, ranging from an asymptomatic lab finding to extremis, the symptoms of hyperglycemia (i.e., **polyuria, polydipsia, blurred vision, fatigue, weight loss**) are usually present. Women frequently present with recurrent vaginal yeast infections.

TREATMENT

How does the goal of therapy differ between type I and type II?	Type I: therapy should focus on insulin replacement; mimicry of normal insulin secretion is the ultimate goal. Type II: therapy focuses on decreasing insulin resistance; insulin administration is used only as a last resort to prevent severe complications of poorly controlled hyperglycemia.
What are the different types of insulin, and how do they differ?	Table 7-2 shows the most commonly used insulin preparations. They vary mostly in terms of pharmacokinetics.

Table 7-2. Pharmacokinetics of Selected Insulin Preparations

Insulin	Peak of Action° (hrs)	Duration of Action° (hrs)
Rapid		
Regular	2–4	6–8
Intermediate		
NPH	6–12	18–24
Lente	6–12	18–24
Long-acting		
Ultralente	18–24	36

° Subcutaneous administration
NPH = neutral protamine Hagedorn

Combination preparations are also available: 70/30 (i.e., 70 units of NPH and 30 units of regular) and 50/50 are the most often used combination preparations.

What is the role of non-insulin therapy in type I DM?

Although eating a healthy diet and exercising regularly helps the type I diabetic by reducing the cardiovascular risk factors, these modalities do not *treat* the diabetes; that is, although the patient needs to adjust the insulin dose to account for diet and exercise, diet and exercise are not treatments for the disease itself. Oral hypoglycemic agents (OHAs) have no role in IDDM.

What is a typical insulin regimen for type I DM?

Insulin regimens will vary widely from patient to patient, but a common approach is a three-shot regimen. The patient uses one daily shot of ultralente to emulate the body's basal production of insulin (0.5–1.0 unit per hour). In addition, the patient uses three shots of regular insulin, which are given before meals and adjusted according to the caloric content of the meal and any exercise plans.

What kind of regimen would a less motivated patient use?

Less educated and less motivated patients often achieve adequate control using a combination of neutral protamine Hagedorn (NPH; insulin) and regular insulin in a two-shot regimen: one shot before breakfast and one before dinner.

What other methods are used to administer insulin to patients with type I DM?

Conversely, extremely tight glucose control can be achieved with an insulin pump, which gives a basal rate of regular insulin subcutaneously with boluses that are programmed to supply insulin for meals. In the future, closed-loop systems that monitor blood glucose and supply insulin as needed might be developed to achieve nearly perfect glycemic control.

What are the treatment modalities for type II DM?

Exercise, diet modifications with weight loss if obese, OHAs, and insulin

What is the role of nonpharmacologic therapy?

The primary treatment goal for type II DM is to reduce insulin resistance and should be attempted initially via:
1. **Diet.** Focus on a reduction of concentrated sweets, saturated fats, and cholesterol, which can effectively reduce blood sugar levels even before significant weight loss is achieved.
2. **Exercise.** It augments weight loss efforts and may also reduce insulin resistance.
   To be effective, these efforts must be explored thoroughly and seriously with the patient. Referral to a nutritionist may be a useful adjunct.

OHAs

What OHAs are available for treatment of DM?

The sulfonylureas and metformin dominate oral therapy.

What are their mechanisms of action?

1. The sulfonylureas—primarily glipizide and glyburide—decrease blood glucose levels by stimulating β cells, increasing insulin production, and stimulating insulin receptors. (**Remember:** These drugs have half-lives up to 30 hours and, in cases of overdose, one must observe patients for a prolonged period to insure against recurrent hypoglycemia.)

2. Metformin, a biguanide that decreases blood glucose levels by reducing intestinal absorption and gluconeogenesis and by increasing glucose use in peripheral tissues. These medicines are frequently used in combination for extra effect.

What are the most common side effects of OHAs?

Sulfonylureas can cause hypoglycemia, which can be profound at times, and is seen most frequently in elderly patients and alcohol abusers. Metformin can cause GI upset.

Insulin Therapy

When should insulin be considered for patients with type I DM?

If diet, exercise, and OHAs do not successfully control blood glucose levels (i.e., fasting blood sugar > 200 mg/dl), insulin is a reasonable adjunct therapy. However, insulin is used in a different manner than insulin replacement therapy in type I DM. In type II DM, giving insulin will actually increase insulin resistance.

What is a reasonable starting regimen of insulin in a patient with type II DM?

Regimens vary based on patient motivation. Common strategies:
1. Usually start with a morning shot of NPH or 70/30 (two thirds of the daily insulin dose) and a second shot (the other one third) in the evening.
2. Less compliant patients may do better with a single daily shot of ultralente.

How can a patient's glycemic control best be monitored?

Capillary blood glucose and glycosylated hemoglobin are commonly used to monitor diabetic control. Glycosylated hemoglobin (as well as hemoglobin A_{1c}) provides a measure of overall glycemic control over the 2–3 months before the test.

How is this information helpful in adjusting their regimen?

It may be especially helpful when short-term conditions (e.g., an infection) are exacerbating control, and the long-term picture is unclear.

Can capillary blood glucose testing be done at home?

Yes. It can be done up to four times daily and is an essential tool in timing, type, and dosage of insulin injections, which vary widely from patient to patient.

Why is home glucose monitoring important?

Although frequency of testing varies widely, depending on the patient's motivation and the severity of their disease, all diabetics should know how to check their blood sugar. Patients on insulin therapy need to follow their sugar at home closely after initiation of a regimen or changes in insulin dose. Patients should also know to check their sugar if they become ill, because new symptoms may reflect a change in sugar or may be a part of a separate process that will cause glycemic instability. For patients unwilling to do this, programs need to be individualized to that patient's needs. Some patients on OHAs may also need to perform home glucose monitoring on a case-by-case basis.

What is the most common complication of insulin therapy?

Hypoglycemia—both alterations in diet and mistakes in insulin administration can lead to it.

How does hypoglycemia present?

Symptoms vary widely, but usually include symptoms of adrenergic excess, such as sweating, tremor, tachycardia, and palpitations. Severe hypoglycemic episodes can present as confusion, mental status changes, or even coma. Treatment with D_{50} should be initiated immediately in any patient with these symptoms, but particularly in a known diabetic.

What is another common side effect of insulin therapy?

Weight gain

What do these various diabetes treatments cost?

Treatment of diabetes with OHAs and insulin can be quite expensive, which is another reason to emphasize diet and exercise as first-line therapy (Table 7–3).

Table 7-3. Cost of Diabetes Agents

Therapy	Amount	Local Cost of 30-Day Supply ($)
Medication		
Glucotrol-XL	10 mg, qd	26.79
Metformin	500 mg, bid	37.69
NPH Insulin	75 U/day (divided doses)	36.00
Supplies		
Test Strips	Use 1, bid	42.00
Syringes, 1 ml	Use 1, bid	6.63

NPH = neutral protamine Hagedorn

COMPLICATIONS OF DIABETES

What are the most common causes of hyperglycemia in a patient with diabetes?

In a stable diabetic, a hyperglycemic episode will often have an identifiable etiology for which the vigilant physician should be alert. Remember the **three I's**—**I**nfection, **I**nflammation, and **I**nfarction—which are the most common precipitants and may not be readily apparent. Administration of glucocorticoids and noncompliance will also cause elevated blood sugars and need to be recognized.

What is diabetic ketoacidosis (DKA)?

DKA is the most common acute cause of death directly attributable to DM. It occurs almost exclusively in type I diabetes, when a sustained period of hyperglycemia leads to an osmotic diuresis and dehydration. At the same time, breakdown of fats to free fatty acids and gluconeogenesis exacerbate the acidosis.

How does DKA present?

Patients will present with severe dehydration and often with nausea, vomiting, and abdominal pain. Kussmaul respirations (fast, deep breaths) develop in an attempt to blow off excess CO_2. The ketones may be apparent as a fruity scent on the patient's breath. Lab tests will show an elevated blood glucose (usually > 400n mg/dl) and a metabolic acidosis with an increased anion gap. Ketones can be detected in both blood and urine.

What is the treatment for DKA?

Treatment is individualized and depends mostly on rehydration and administration of insulin, usually by way of an IV drip. In addition, one must be vigilant about replacement of depleted electrolytes, particularly potassium and phosphate.

What parameters should be followed during the treatment of DKA?

pH should be followed directly with serial ABGs, and venous sampling should be done until the anion gap has returned to normal.

How does one calculate the anion gap?

Anion gap = $Na - (Cl + HCO_3)$. Normal values are $< 12 (\pm 2)$.

What is nonketotic hyperosmolar syndrome?

Occurring most often in type II DM patients, this condition is typified by severe dehydration, extreme hyperglycemia (usually > 600 mg/dl), hyperosmolarity, and mental status changes. Acidosis, which is prevented by residual insulin activity, is not a feature of this syndrome.

How is this syndrome treated?

Treatment is similar to that for DKA, but morbidity and mortality are high, and care must be taken to lower the osmolarity slowly to prevent undue cerebral edema.

What are the long-term consequences of diabetes?

Perhaps the most common and most alarming complications of DM arise from the vasculopathies. Microvascular disease affects the eye and the kidney. Macrovascular disease leads to arteriosclerosis, causing heart attacks, strokes, and severe peripheral vascular disease at a young age. Neuropathies also devastate these patients, with peripheral neuropathy, impotence, and incontinence, frequently developing after many years. Together, these processes predispose diabetics to foot ulcers, polymicrobial infections that evade treatment, and often lead to amputations.

What are the two types of diabetic retinopathy?

Nonproliferative (NPR) and proliferative retinopathy

Describe NPR.

NPR, found in nearly all diabetics after 25 years of having the disease, is comprised of background changes (microaneurysms, cotton-wool spots, and retinal hemorrhages) that usually do not affect vision.

Describe proliferative diabetic retinopathy.

It rarely occurs and consists of neovascularization, which can threaten visual acuity. It can be controlled with photocoagulation and should be detected early. Similarly, cataracts and glaucoma are more common in DM.

How should diabetic retinopathy be followed?

Recommendations currently include annual ophthalmologic examination for all diabetics of more than 5 years (**Remember:** it is difficult to know when type II DM starts, because it is frequently diagnosed after an extended period).

How should the primary care physician screen for and treat early diabetic nephropathy in type II diabetics?

Data show that detection of microalbuminuria and treatment with captopril can slow progression to albuminuria (> 300 mg/dl). In type I patients, treatment of albuminuria with captopril led to decreased mortality and slowed progression to renal failure. However, there are no data regarding type II patients and progression of renal disease. Therefore, it is reasonable to dip urine once or twice per year to check for protein. If a diabetic dips positive for protein, treatment with an ACE inhibitor is indicated. Referral to a nephrologist is appropriate when the creatinine surpasses 3 mg/dl. Additional data suggest that good blood sugar control (Gly Hgb ≈ 7%–8%) retards progression of renal disease.

How will worsening renal failure affect glycemic control?

Because insulin is cleared by the kidney, worsening renal failure can decrease excretion of insulin and lead to potentially dangerous hypoglycemia. This should be suspected when a long-time diabetic has an "improvement" in glycemic control without other explanation.

How can diabetic patients reduce their risk from macrovascular disease?

Control of other cardiovascular risk factors is paramount in these patients. Smoking cessation, weight loss, activity, and control of hypertension take on much greater importance.

How may the symptoms of macrovascular disease differ in the diabetic?

Symptoms of coronary artery disease (CAD), as well as other symptoms of other vasculopathies can be greatly mitigated by a coincident neuropathy. Silent myocardial ischemia and infarct can be difficult to diagnose and should always be on the differential diagnosis in these high-risk patients.

How may treatments differ?

Treatment of vascular disease, especially in the extremities, is much more difficult in diabetics who have more diffuse lesions and poorer healing capacity.

How tightly should diabetics control their diabetes?

This is the central question that has troubled family physicians and endocrinologist for years, and unfortunately the debate has not been settled. In 1993, the DCCT trial showed that in IDDM patients' tight glycemic control (Gly Hgb ≈ 7%) led to improvement in several disease-oriented, intermediate outcomes. However, it also led to an increase in severe episodes of hypoglycemia. No data were collected regarding patient-oriented outcomes, such as death and renal failure; no data of this type exist on type II diabetics.

All agree that glycemic control should be sufficient to ward off hyperglycemic symptoms and DKA (Gly Hgb < 10%) but, beyond this, further efforts need to be individualized. The tradeoff between more frequent hypoglycemic episodes and a potential decrease in long-term complications should be explored with the patient and the rigor of therapy based on the shared value judgment that emerges from that discussion.

Within the next year, a 20-year cohort of type II diabetics will be published, which mirrors the DCCT in design but also looks at mortality and patient-oriented outcomes. These results may greatly influence the way primary care physicians care for their diabetic patients.

THYROID DISEASE

What is the most physiologically active thyroid hormone?

Triiodothyronine (T_3)

What is the pathway by which it is produced?

Twenty percent of T_3 is produced directly in the thyroid gland, and 80% comes from extrathyroidal deiodination of thyroxine (T_4).

How is the production of active thyroid hormones regulated by the body?

A negative feedback loop between both T_3 and T_4 and the hypothalamic–pituitary axis controls hormone production. Thyroid-stimulating hormone (TSH) and thyrotropin-releasing hormone (TRH) are intermediate actors in this path.

Which laboratory test is most useful in assessing thyroid function?

TSH level—in the absence of hypothalamic–pituitary disease, the TSH will accurately reflect the body's thyroid state by showing whether the feedback loop is trying to rev up or slow down T_4 production

What is measured by the T_3 uptake?

Not to be confused with a radioactive iodine uptake study, this is an in vitro assay that measures the uptake of radioactively labeled T_3 by available thyroid-binding sites. The resulting value is an indirect measure of unoccupied T_4-binding globulin (TBG) sites.

HYPERTHYROIDISM

A 43-year-old woman presents with weight loss (although with a good appetite), diarrhea, and the complaint of "feeling hot all the time." What is the most likely diagnosis?	This is a classic presentation of hyperthyroidism (thyrotoxicosis).
What additional history and physical findings would confirm this?	History: nervousness, heart palpitations, emotional instability, or menstrual irregularities Physical findings: an enlarged thyroid gland, thyroid bruit, fine tremor, tachycardia or atrial fibrillation, nail changes (Plummer's nails), and brisk reflexes (decreased relaxation phase)
What is the most common cause of hyperthyroidism?	Graves' disease—an autoimmune disorder that presents as thyrotoxicosis with an enlarged thyroid and characteristic ophthalmopathy
What are other common causes of hyperthyroidism?	Toxic multinodular goiter, thyroiditis, and factitious thyrotoxicosis Rare but important etiologies include pituitary adenoma, ovarian cancer, or primary thyroid carcinoma.
What is Graves' ophthalmopathy?	This infiltrative process varies in severity from lid lag to proptosis to extraocular muscle involvement to effects on the cornea or optic nerve. It may correlate to the severity of thyroid dysfunction and may resolve with treatment of the thyroid abnormalities.
Given a patient with symptoms of hyperthyroidism, an increased T_4, and a decreased TSH, how can the differential diagnosis of hyperthyroidism be investigated?	1. **Physical exam** may be a helpful starting point. Graves' disease usually presents with a bilaterally enlarged gland, frequently accompanied by a bruit. Subacute thyroiditis may also present with an enlarged gland, which tends to be more tender. A multinodular goiter should be

palpable as such, and a solitary functioning nodule may also be palpable.

2. **Radioactive iodine uptake assay** may be helpful if the etiology remains unclear. Uptake will be high in Graves' disease, as in toxic nodules or an adenoma. Uptake is typically low in thyroiditis.

What is a free T_4 (FT_4) index, and when is it useful?

The FT_4 is calculated as:

$$T_3 \text{ uptake} \times \text{total } T_4$$

It adjusts the T_4 value for conditions that may alter the number of thyroid-binding sites, such as pregnancy, nephrotic syndrome, and drugs (e.g., phenytoin, birth control pills).

What is the treatment of choice for hyperthyroidism due to Graves' disease?

The goal is to stop the thyroid gland's overproduction of thyroid hormone and to titrate replacement of T_4 with exogenous hormone. Currently, the two methods are:

1. **Radioablation with ^{131}I:** the preferred modality (but is unacceptable in pregnant women and in children)

2. **Suppression with an antithyroid agent,** such as propylthiouracil (PTU) or methimazole

What is thyroid storm, and how does it present?

Thyroid storm, or severe, acute thyrotoxicosis, is often precipitated by an extreme stressor and usually presents with tachycardia, hypertension, and fever. It is life-threatening, and heart failure and arrhythmias are common.

What is the immediate treatment?

PTU and β-blockade, as well as glucocorticoids, if indicated.

What is the primary toxicity of PTU?

Agranulocytosis may occur in 0.4% of patients and is usually reversible with discontinuation of the medication. It is helpful to get a baseline WBC count before initiating therapy.

HYPOTHYROIDISM

What are the common presenting signs and symptoms of hypothyroidism?

Cold intolerance, weight gain, fatigue, constipation, and drying and thinning of the skin

What are the physical exam findings?

Physical exam reveals hypothermia, bradycardia, and slowing of the relaxation phase of deep tendon reflexes. In addition, hypothyroidism must always be considered in the evaluation of depressive mood disorders and dementia.

What is myxedema?

The extreme presentation of decreased thyroid function. Deposition of a protein/mucopolysaccharide fluid into the tissues gives the patient a doughy appearance. Internal deposition can lead to a pericardial effusion (and subsequent tamponade) or hypoventilation secondary to respiratory muscle involvement. Myxedema coma and myxedema madness represent the rare but dangerous endpoints of this illness.

What is congenital hypothyroidism?

Inadequate thyroid hormone production from birth; this condition rapidly causes mental retardation and developmental delay; it is part of newborn screening programs in most states.

Iatrogenic causes notwithstanding, what is the most common cause of hypothyroidism?

Hashimoto's thyroiditis, an autoimmune disease, leads to decreased hormone production secondary to a synthesis defect.

When replacing thyroid hormone, with what dose should one begin?

In general, it is safe to begin patients at 0.05 mg/day of L-thyroxine.

What comorbidities need to be considered?

CAD is a primary concern. If present, consider starting the dose at 0.025 mg/day. (**Remember:** "Start low and go slow" is the rule, because it is rarely urgent to achieve a euthyroid state.)

HYPERLIPIDEMIA AND HYPERCHOLESTEROLEMIA

What is hyperlipidemia?

Hyperlipidemia is an elevation in plasma cholesterol level and/or plasma triglyceride level.

What specific changes are concerning to the primary care physician?

There is an association between high LDL cholesterol levels and the incidence of CAD. Similarly, low levels of HDL cholesterol have also been associated with an increase in heart disease.

What is the prevalence of hyperlipidemia in the general population?

Sources vary in exact number, but probably 20%–30% of the United States population suffer from this abnormality.

What physical exam finding might tip off the clinician to a hyperlipidemic state?

Tuberous xanthomas and/or a corneal arcus are signs of a significantly elevated lipid state.

What hyperlipidemias are commonly seen in everyday primary care practice?

Type II (elevated LDL)
Type IIa (elevated LDL and triglycerides)
Type IV (elevated triglycerides)

What medical conditions can lead to secondary hyperlipidemia?

Diabetes mellitus, obesity, hypothyroidism, chronic renal disease, and use of thiazide diuretics and β-blockers can all increase plasma lipid levels. Estrogens and alcohol can significantly increase triglyceride levels.

What condition can be precipitated by high triglyceride levels?

Acute pancreatitis

What are the current National Cholesterol Education Program (NCEP) recommendations for the treatment of hypercholesterolemia?

The NCEP issued the following guidelines in 1993. [**Note:** These guidelines are derived from expert opinion and are not entirely consistent with the available evidence on the efficacy of drugs in the treatment of hyperlipidemia (*JAMA* 1993;269;3015)]. The guidelines are based on LDL cholesterol levels and the presence of other risk factors for CAD:

1. **Dietary therapy** should be initiated for:

   Low-risk patients with LDL > 160
   High-risk patients with LDL >130
   Very high-risk patients with LDL > 100

2. **Drug treatment** is considered for use only after 6 months of diet and exercise have been unsuccessful for:

   Low-risk patients with LDL > 190–220
   High-risk patients with LDL > 160
   Very high-risk patients with LDL > 100

What are the principles used in dietary treatment of hypercholesterolemia?

1. Limit fat intake: to < 30% (and < 10% of saturated fat) of total caloric intake
2. Decrease cholesterol: to < 300 mg/day (A more restrictive diet is reserved for those who fail to achieve results after 90 days.)
3. Additional goals: increasing intake of bran, beans, fruits, and vegetables; weight loss

What drugs are considered first-line therapy for hypercholesterolemia?

The HMG CoA reductase inhibitors are now the most popular choice for this condition. Lovastatin, simvastatin, and pravastatin are effective in decreasing LDL cholesterol levels by 30%–50% and increasing HDL cholesterol levels by 5%–10%.

What are the principal side effects?

Myositis and GI upset are common. Because these drugs can significantly increase liver enzymes, the physician should follow them closely.

What other drugs have traditionally been used to treat elevated cholesterol, and what are their effects?

Niacin decreases LDL by 15%–20% and triglycerides by 25%–35%. Colestipol and cholestyramine can decrease LDL by 30% with a slight increase in HDL.

In terms of decreasing the overall mortality, what do the data show as the effectiveness of drug treatment of hypercholesterolemia?

This may strike some as an odd question, given the nearly unanimous medical opinion on this matter and the zeal with which many physicians present their beliefs, but little data are currently available on this most important fact.

Out of over 25 studies that have looked at overall mortality, only two large, double-blind, placebo-controlled studies provide convincing data that drug treatment of hypercholesterolemia reduces overall mortality.

The Simvastatin Scandinavian Survival Study (4S) showed a decrease in total mortality of 30% when simvastatin was given to men with a known history of CAD (secondary prevention). As for primary prevention of heart disease, in the West of Scotland Study, pravastatin was given to a cohort of men with hypercholesterolemia but without known CAD. The result was a 30% decrease in mortality, but unfortunately the result was not quite statistically significant, with a p-value of 0.051 (A p-value of $<$ 0.05 is generally accepted as significant).

How do we treat hypercholesterolemia in an uncertain world?

Many doctors use the HMG CoA reductase inhibitors freely, quite convinced of the intermediate (disease-oriented) data and unwilling to wait for more definitive mortality (patient-oriented) data to arrive. Others will use pravastatin for primary prevention and simvastatin for secondary prevention, citing the above studies and eschewing the other drugs where no data exist. Still others remain skeptical and will cite the paucity of data (particularly in women and heterogeneous populations). These doctors will have a significantly higher threshold to use these medicines. Most certainly, as financial constraints creep closer to the treatment room, this is an issue that will fuel heated debate and, hopefully, a clearer picture of the costs and benefits of treatment.

8   Common Gastrointestinal Problems

APPENDICITIS

What is it?	Inflammation of the vermiform appendix
What causes it?	The initiating event(s) that precipitate appendicitis is unclear. Although obstruction of the appendix by a fecalith has been observed, this is not a consistent finding. Regardless, an inflammatory response is initiated and leads to edema, swelling, and ischemia of the appendix. If not removed, the appendix will eventually necrose and rupture.
What complications can occur if appendicitis is not promptly recognized and treated?	Rupture, abscess, diffuse peritonitis, sepsis, shock, and death
What are common symptoms of appendicitis?	Abdominal pain, anorexia, nausea, and vomiting are the initial symptoms of appendicitis. Fever, chills, and dizziness follow if not diagnosed and treated promptly.
What are the classic characteristics of abdominal pain with appendicitis?	The pain begins in the periumbilical region and moves to the right lower quadrant as the process progresses.
What are common physical findings of appendicitis?	1. Diminished or absent bowel sounds are the most common findings 2. Low-grade fever

3. Tenderness and pain: abdominal tenderness in the right lower quadrant (especially at McBurney's point); tenderness on the right side of the rectum during digital exam and pain with flexion and internal rotation of the hip (psoas sign) can indicate an inflamed retrocecal appendix.

What are less common findings?

Pain with abrupt movement (e.g., bumping the exam table, jumping from the exam table to the floor), high fever, and hypotension are less common and found with diffuse peritoneal irritation, such as with rupture of the appendix.

Where is McBurney's point?

The point on the right lower abdomen that is halfway between the anterior–superior iliac crest and the umbilicus.

What diagnostic tests are used, and what findings indicate appendicitis?

White blood count (WBC) is initially elevated to a mild-to-moderate degree ($12,000–15,000/mm^3$). As symptoms progress, the WBC continues to rise. A very high WBC is indicative of rupture and/or abscess.

Abdominal ultrasound. An enlarged, edematous appendix on ultrasound is a reliable diagnostic finding. However, ultrasound is not a reliable diagnostic test if the appendix is not well visualized (i.e., if the appendix is not visualized, it does not indicate that the appendix is normal).

Abdominal CT is better at distinguishing a normal from an abnormal appendix, but still cannot identify abnormal appendices in all cases (especially early appendicitis).

How is appendicitis treated?

Surgical removal of the appendix is the treatment of choice, preferably before it ruptures. The procedure is frequently performed via the laparoscopy with minimal morbidity.

What are the admission criteria?

1. All patients undergoing appendectomy

2. Patients with suspected appendicitis in which clinical suspicion is not high enough to indicate surgery, but indicative of observation and surgical consultation
3. Patients with suspected appendiceal rupture or abscess

Helpful hints

1. Surgical consultation is indicated early if appendicitis is suspected. Surgical input can be helpful when the clinical picture is unclear.
2. Appendicitis is still mainly a clinical diagnosis. Surgery is indicated on all patients with a high clinical suspicion of appendicitis even if other diagnostic tests are normal. To attempt to remove all inflamed appendices before they rupture, some normal appendices are removed. The rate of removal of normal appendices should be around 10%. If the surgeon's rate is higher than that, he/she may operate too quickly. If it is significantly lower, the surgeon may not operate quickly enough.

CONSTIPATION

What is it?

The subjective feeling of needing to pass stool but being unable to do so

What causes it?

The most common cause is hard stool caused by inadequate dietary intake of fiber and water. Other causes can include autonomic dysfunction leading to impaired peristalsis, obstruction from tumor, laxative overuse/abuse, physical inactivity, drugs that impair peristalsis, and/or advancing age.

What patients are at high risk for constipation?

Inactive, elderly patients with multiple medical problems and multidrug regimens

Diabetic patients, who are at increased risk for autonomic dysfunction and impaired peristalsis

Patients with poor dietary habits or insufficient resources to maintain adequate dietary fiber

What other symptoms are commonly associated with constipation?

Abdominal bloating and/or distention
Flatulence
Rectal pain with defecation
Excessive straining to pass stools
Loose stools (caused by passing liquid stool around hard stool that won't pass)

What are common physical findings with constipation?

Distended, minimally tender abdomen that is tympanitic to percussion
Sometimes hard stool can be palpated in the left paracolic gutter in the outer/lower edge of the left lower quadrant.
Rectal exam frequently finds large amounts of hard stool in the rectal vault.

What diagnostic tests are used?

Occult blood testing on stool from rectal exam can indicate blood loss from polyp or tumor. Plain radiograph of the abdomen can show stool filling the rectum and/or colon. Barium enema or colonoscopy can be used but are usually not necessary to make the diagnosis.

How is constipation treated?

1. Ingesting adequate fiber (e.g., by increasing fruits, vegetables, and whole grain cereal products into diet) and water is the key to treatment in most cases. Ingesting fiber without adequate water is a common mistake made by persons with constipation and will make it worse.
2. Stool-bulking agents add fiber in a non-food form.
3. Stool softeners retain more water to provide a stool that passes easier.
4. Laxatives stimulate peristalsis to propel stool from the rectum.
5. Mineral oils lubricate the stool and stimulate peristalsis.
6. Suppositories and enemas stimulate, lubricate, and/or distend the rectum (depending on the agent used) to get hard, impacted stool to pass.

How is constipation prevented?

Regularly review the patient's dietary intake of fiber and water, especially in patients at increased risk. Regular exercise is also important to avoid constipation. Ask about any difficulty passing stool as part of health maintenance; identifying the problem early may help prevent severe problems.

What are complications of constipation?

Hemorrhoids and diverticular disease are secondary to the increased pressures created by straining at stool. Fecal impaction with partial or total obstruction occur from large, hard stools that accumulate in the rectal vault and can't pass through the anal sphincter.

What are the admission criteria?

Fecal impaction causing obstruction in a person who is physically unable to perform needed treatments (e.g., enemas, suppositories, frequent trips to the bathroom) and does not have adequate support from family or friends to accomplish treatment, although this is rare

Helpful hints

1. Patients with long-standing constipation often need a bowel regimen (combination of agents used regularly) to prevent impaction.
2. Patients are often hesitant to discuss bowel habits. You should initiate the discussion.

DIARRHEA

What is it?

Passing liquid or very loose, semisolid stool

What causes it?

GI infection, parasitic infestation, bleeding, ischemia, inflammatory bowel disease (IBD), fecal impaction, anxiety, malabsorption, and drugs; previous surgical resection of significant portions of the stomach or small or large intestine can also result in diarrhea

What historical factors help distinguish etiology?

The length of onset and duration of symptoms distinguish acute diarrhea (usually infectious) from chronic diarrhea.

What symptoms are commonly associated with diarrhea?

Nausea, vomiting, fever, abdominal bloating and/or pain, rectal pain, mucus or blood in stool, melena (black, tarry stool), thirst, and decreased urinary frequency

What physical findings are commonly associated with diarrhea?

Mild, diffuse abdominal tenderness is the most common finding. Dry mucous membranes with postural hypotension and poor skin turgor indicate significant dehydration. Melena or frank blood in the stool indicates significant GI bleeding. Occult blood may have multiple causes (e.g., irritation from some infectious agents, inflammatory disease). Weight loss with wasting of muscle mass can indicate malnutrition from chronic malabsorption.

What diagnostic tests are performed?

1. Gross observation of the stool for blood, melena, and so on
2. Microscopic evaluation with appropriate stains for WBCs, parasites, and their ova
3. Occult blood testing
4. Bacterial cultures
5. Colonoscopy if inflammatory disease or significant bleeding is suspected in the lower GI tract

What are common infectious agents that cause diarrhea?

Viral gastroenteritis is the most common cause of diarrhea in the United States. Bacteria and parasites are also fairly common causes of diarrhea and gastroenteritis.

What are the most common bacteria that cause diarrhea?

Salmonella, Shigella, and *Campylobacter* species; toxigenic *Escherichia coli*

Do antibiotics help patients with bacterial diarrhea?

Yes and no. *Campylobacter* and toxigenic *E. coli* are treated with antibiotics but are not as common as *Salmonella* or *Shigella*. *Salmonella* and *Shigella* infections are self-limited and do not require antibiotics. Treating *Salmonella* infections with antibiotics can actually be harmful, because it prolongs the carrier state.

What are common parasitic infections that cause diarrhea?

Giardia lamblia is the most common organism in immune competent hosts. *Cryptosporidium* and other parasites can occur but are more common in immunocompromised hosts.

How is diarrhea treated?

The most effective treatment is to treat the underlying etiology, if possible. However, because the most common cause of diarrhea (viral infection) has no specific treatment, the most important treatment issue is to prevent the patient from dehydrating. Hypotonic solutions of water with carbohydrate and small amounts of sodium and potassium are recommended for oral rehydration. Sodas and sports drinks should be avoided, because they are hyperosmolar and can exacerbate fluid loss. Significant dehydration may require IV rehydration (especially in children). Agents that impair GI motility should be used with caution. They can prolong diarrhea secondary to infection and can increase complications in *Salmonella* infections (thus they should be avoided in these cases). However, they can be helpful and used safely in patients with anxiety or malabsorption.

What are the most effective methods of preventing diarrhea?

1. Infectious agents that cause diarrhea are very contagious. Patients in adult or child day-care centers or those who work in these facilities are at high risk for acquiring these infections.
2. Appropriately cooking meats can prevent most infections with bacterial agents (e.g., toxigenic *E. coli*, *Salmonella*) that can have serious complications (GI mucosal invasion, sepsis, death).
3. The single most important public health advance in the twentieth century is the development of systems that provide clean, safe drinking water. In developed countries, this has eliminated what was previously the number one cause of mortality in children—diarrheal illness.

What are the admission criteria for a patient with diarrhea?	1. Significant dehydration (e.g., poor skin turgor, decreased urinary output, hypotension), especially in someone with continued vomiting 2. Continued bleeding, bleeding from unknown source, blood loss requiring transfusion 3. Malabsorption associated with malnutrition and weight loss requiring parenteral hyperalimentation

CHOLELITHIASIS

What is it?	The formation of stones in the gallbladder
What is the composition of gallstones?	Ninety percent of stones are cholesterol and 10% are calcium.
What causes gallstones?	An excessive concentration of cholesterol or calcium accumulates in the bile stored in the gallbladder and leads to the formation of precipitates, which are known as *stones*.
What is the classic presentation of cholelithiasis?	Transient, recurrent right upper quadrant abdominal pain (colicky pain), nausea and/or vomiting, especially 30–40 minutes after a fatty meal, is the classic presentation.
What are less common complaints?	Less common complaints include anorexia, persistent pain, abdominal bloating, light-colored stool, dark (tea-colored) urine, and right upper back or shoulder pain (referred pain).
What does the colicky pain correlate with?	Movement of the stone through the common bile and hepatic duct; the pain ceases when the stone passes through the sphincter of Oddi and into the duodenum
What are common physical findings with cholecystitis?	Right upper quadrant or epigastric tenderness is the most common finding, although the exam may be completely normal between episodes. Murphy's sign is a classic finding.
What is Murphy's sign?	Deep palpation of the right upper quadrant just below the costal margin as

the patient inhales causes the patient acute pain; on palpation, the patient ceases the inspiratory effort and exhales because of the acute pain.

What laboratory diagnostic tests are used?

Urinalysis, serum bilirubin, serum amylase, and liver enzymes

What radiographic tests are used?

Gallbladder ultrasound, oral cholecystogram (OCG), and/or abdominal CT are common radiological studies

What laboratory findings would increase likelihood of cholecystitis?
   Serum bilirubin?

Hepatic dysfunction from altered bilirubin processing may cause bilirubin in urine and elevated serum levels.

   Serum amylase?

Amylase elevation could indicate pancreatitis from a stone obstructing the common bile duct distal to the insertion of the pancreatic duct.

   Liver enzymes?

Liver enzymes may be elevated from the same process.

What radiographic findings would increase likelihood of cholecystitis?
   Ultrasound?

Ultrasound is the most frequently used diagnostic test. It shows stones (may be small stones that layer or one or more large stones) in the dependent side of the gallbladder as well as obstruction of ducts.

   OCG?

OCG identifies the type of stones (calcium stones are radiodense on the scout film; cholesterol stones are identified with visualization of the gallbladder by oral contrast material) as well as the functional status of the gallbladder (non-visualization by contrast indicates a non-functioning gallbladder).

   CT?

CT can identify stones that are not visualized by the other radiologic tests.

What is the pharmacologic treatment for cholelithiasis?

Oral ursodiol—a six-month regimen leads to resorption of cholesterol stones in most cases

What are special considerations before using ursodiol?

For ursodiol to work, the stones must be small and must consist of cholesterol salts, and the gallbladder must function properly. Therefore, an OCG is required before initiating therapy.

What is the recurrence rate after cessation of Ursodiol?

85%

What is the surgical treatment of cholelithiasis?

Cholecystectomy (i.e., surgical removal of the gallbladder) eliminates stones and their source. It is performed in most cases of symptomatic cholecystitis. Laparoscopic technique minimizes morbidity and time lost from work.

What are the limitations of laparoscopic cholecystectomy?

The major limitation is the inability to evaluate the common bile and cystic ducts for stones. Therefore, endoscopic retrograde cholangiopancreatography (ERCP) is indicated to evaluate the ducts for stones. If stones are found in the ducts, removal is attempted by basket extraction through the endoscope. If this is unsuccessful, the laparoscopic technique is abandoned and an open procedure is indicated.

What are the complications of cholecystitis?

1. Acute, suppurative cholecystitis caused by **obstruction** of the cystic duct by a stone is a medical emergency with high morbidity and mortality from septic complications. Avoiding this complication is the justification given for cholecystectomy in patients with minimal symptoms.
2. **Liver dysfunction** caused by obstruction or infection and pancreatitis caused by obstruction of the common bile duct distal to the insertion of the hepatic duct can also occur. Rarely, small-bowel obstruction can occur from a large stone that passes into the duodenum through a cholecystenteric fistula (gallstone ileus).

What are the admission criteria?	Fever, hypotension, or other evidence of acute suppurative cholecystitis Pancreatitis or moderate-to-severe hepatic dysfunction Intractable vomiting Patients requiring IV rehydration or parenteral pain control in anticipation of surgery
Helpful hints	1. Medical therapy with ursodiol can be especially helpful in patients who are poor surgical risks. 2. There is no evidence that outcomes are improved with surgery in asymptomatic or minimally symptomatic patients despite the concern of potential complications.

GASTROESOPHAGEAL REFLUX DISEASE (GERD)

What is it?	It is a clinical syndrome with symptoms secondary to the reflux of gastric contents into the esophagus, larynx, and/or pharynx. Symptoms and complications are caused by the low pH of gastric secretions irritating the mucosal surfaces they contact.
How does this differ from vomiting?	GERD is not associated with forceful gastric contraction and expulsion of contents as is seen with vomiting. The refluxed material is usually liquid and relatively small in volume.
What causes GERD?	Lower esophageal sphincter (LES) dysfunction is the primary cause of GERD. It is often associated with or exacerbated by hiatal hernia, obesity, and drugs that lower LES pressure. Esophageal motility disorders from autonomic nervous dysfunction or infiltrating diseases (e.g., scleroderma, lymphoma) also cause GERD.
What three commonly used substances lower LES pressure?	Alcohol, caffeine, and nicotine

What are common symptoms of GERD?

Heartburn (i.e., burning chest pain)
Epigastric pain
Water brash (tasting bitter fluid in the mouth or throat)
Cough

What aggravates symptoms?

Symptoms are exacerbated by maneuvers that increase gastric pressure (e.g., tight clothing, consuming a large meal) or change the force of gravity acting on stomach contents (e.g., lying down).

What are common physical findings of GERD?

Usually the physical exam is normal. However, in some cases, mild epigastric tenderness, reproduction of symptoms with epigastric pressure, erythema of the pharynx, and/or dental decay caused by reflux are found.

What are four tests that may be used for diagnosing GERD?

1. Upper endoscopy
2. Barium esophagogram
3. Esophageal pH monitoring
4. Esophageal manometry

What findings on these tests indicate GERD?
Upper endoscopy?

The advantage of endoscopy is that the mucosa can be visualized and biopsies can be performed to evaluate for complications. The disadvantage is that results may be normal in up to 50% of patients with GERD (i.e., low negative predictive value). Endoscopy is best for patients with persistent symptoms unresponsive to empiric medical therapy or for patients with symptoms of complications.

Barium esophagogram?

Because it reproduces the physiology of eating, it can be helpful in identifying esophageal motility problems. It can also identify aspiration or stricture. Unfortunately, as with endoscopy, its negative predictive value is low.

Esophageal pH monitoring?

It can correlate pH changes with symptoms, identifying reflux in patients with atypical symptoms, and document pH levels in patients unresponsive to treatment. It is not indicated in most patients.

Esophageal manometry?

It documents adequacy of esophageal peristalsis and LES pressure. Unfortunately, these measurements do not correlate well with symptoms or predict success of therapy. It is not indicated in most patients.

How is GERD treated?

The first line of therapy is a combination of lifestyle modifications and OTC antacids. When these fail, medical therapy is generally successful in reducing symptoms and/or treating complications. Rarely, surgery is indicated in patients with complications despite aggressive medical therapy.

What lifestyle modifications are used?

The patient should avoid substances that lower LES pressure (e.g., alcohol, caffeine, nicotine). Loose clothing, weight loss, small meals, avoiding eating close to bedtime, and raising the head of the bed on bricks counteract the factors (e.g., increased gastric pressure and lack of gravity) that make symptoms worse and can help alleviate symptoms.

What are the general principles of medical therapy of GERD?

Medications are used to increase LES pressure, improve esophageal and gastric peristalsis, raise gastric pH, and decrease the volume of gastric secretions.

What are the two general classes of drugs, examples of each class, and their mechanism of action?

1. **Drugs that increase gastric pH and decrease volume of secretions.** Decreasing acidity eliminates or greatly decreases the irritant effect of refluxed material and, therefore, improves or eliminates symptoms. Decreased acidity is accomplished by decreasing acid secretion, which also decreases volume of gastric secretions. H_2 receptor antagonists (cimetidine, ranitidine) and proton pump inhibitors (omeprazole) fall into this category and have been shown to be 70%–90% effective.
2. **Promotility agents,** which are drugs that increase LES pressure and

promote esophageal peristalsis and gastric emptying. Metoclopramide and cisapride are the most frequently used agents that are effective in decreasing symptoms.

What are some complications of GERD?

Erosive esophagitis
Esophageal stricture formation
Barrett's esophagus
Esophageal cancer
Chronic hoarseness
Chronic cough and asthma

What are the admission criteria for a patient with GERD?

Patients with simple GERD almost never require hospitalization. Only severe complications (e.g., malnutrition caused by stricture, cancer that requires parenteral hyperalimentation and/or surgery) require admission.

Helpful hints

1. **Proton pump inhibitors** are effective for symptom control and treatment of erosive esophagitis. Laboratory rats have developed gastrin-secreting tumors with prolonged use, but this has not been observed in humans with up to five years of continuous usage. Discussing this issue with the patient and periodic monitoring of gastrin levels are recommended by some if long-term use of these agents is planned.

2. **Empiric medical therapy** is indicated for patients with reflux and no symptoms of complications. Further evaluation is indicated if the patient does not respond to treatment.

3. **Fundoplication surgery** can be 85% effective in eliminating symptoms but the fundoplication usually breaks down over time.

COLON CANCER

What is it?

Cancer of the large intestine

What is the most frequent histologic type?

Adenocarcinoma

What causes it?

The only known direct cause is genetic: familial polyposis; Lynch syndromes I and II are autosomal dominant genetic conditions in which colon cancer occurs at a young age

What, other than the familial syndromes, are risk factors for colon cancer?

Increasing age (90% occur in persons > 50 years of age)
High fat–low fiber diet
Family history of colon cancer that is not a documented genetic syndrome
Severe IBD

What are common symptoms of colon cancer?

Early in the course of colon cancer, the patient will have no symptoms. As the lesion progresses, mild symptoms (e.g., constipation, cramping, mild pain and/or blood on or in the stool) can occur. Advanced lesions can cause anorexia, weight loss, frank bleeding, and/or obstruction.

What are common physical findings in colon cancer?

The most common finding is occult blood in the stool on testing but this can be variable. A rectal or abdominal mass can sometimes be found and metastatic disease can cause hepatomegaly or jaundice.

What diagnostic tests are used to identify colon cancer?

CBC and serum chemistries can detect anemia, impaired nutrition (low albumin), and elevated transaminases (elevated with metastatic disease) that are frequently associated with colon cancer. Barium enema can detect most significant lesions and identify some polyps. Colonoscopy with biopsy not only can obtain tissue for definitive diagnosis but can detect other lesions (e.g., polyps, cancers) that may need treatment.

Is a rectal exam a useful screening tool?

There is no evidence that rectal exam is useful in screening for colon cancer. At present, no evidence-based screening strategies recommend its use for this purpose.

How is colon cancer treated?

Surgical removal of the tumor and adjacent colon with or without

chemotherapy, depending on the stage
of the lesion

**What are the most
important ambulatory care
issues for colon cancer?**

Early detection and/or prevention

**What tests are used to
detect asymptomatic
cancers and/or
precancerous polyps?**

Occult blood testing of stools and/or
flexible sigmoidoscopy

How often is each done?

Recommendation is to perform occult
blood testing yearly on three stool
samples, and flexible sigmoidoscopy is
recommended at five-year intervals.
Although there is evidence that using
these tests saves lives, the optimum time
frame and combination of these tests are
unclear.

**What is the next step if
either of these tests is
positive?**

Colonoscopy

**What are the admission
criteria?**

Dehydration, malnutrition and/or anemia
requiring parenteral fluids,
hyperalimentation or blood products,
respectively. Active rectal bleeding,
hepatic impairment, or intestinal
obstruction may also require admission.
It is essential to involve the patient in all
treatment decisions so that disease
severity and prognosis can be considered
before costly treatments that may
prolong life, but not improve quality, are
used.

Helpful hints

1. Significant controversies still exist
   regarding the optimum approach for
   screening for colon cancer. An open
   mind to new data is essential to
   develop an evidence-based approach
   to colon cancer screening.
2. Intestinal obstruction is a painful
   condition and surgical intervention
   should be considered even in
   terminal patients.

3. Advance directives and end-of-life issues need to be discussed and reviewed.
4. Pain control is imperative in all terminally ill patients. Do not hesitate to use narcotics in these patients, if needed.

HEMORRHOIDS

What is a hemorrhoid?

A dilated vein (varicose vein) at the external edge (external hemorrhoid) or internal edge (internal hemorrhoid) of the anal sphincter.

What causes it?

Increased venous pressure exceeds the elasticity of the vessel wall, causing a ballooning of the wall of the vessel. This can occur with straining at stool, pregnancy, or medical conditions that increase portal vein pressure (e.g., cirrhosis).

What are common symptoms of hemorrhoids?

Rectal pain and itching, blood on the stool or toilet paper, blood in the toilet bowl

What are common physical findings?

Dilated venous protrusions around or protruding from the anus. The hemorrhoid may contain clotted blood (thrombosed hemorrhoid) or bleed from a tear or abrasion of the surface. Hemorrhoids protruding from above are usually internal hemorrhoids.

What diagnostic tests are used?

Usually, physical exam is all that is needed. Flexible sigmoidoscopy, colonoscopy, or barium enema can be considered if significant rectal bleeding or anemia is present.

How are hemorrhoids treated?

1. Softening the stool (i.e., increasing fiber and water in the diet with or without stool softeners), sitz baths, and anesthetic creams or ointments with or without hydrocortisone are initial treatments.

2. Using moist wipes rather than toilet paper can also decrease itching and irritation. Baby wipes are inexpensive and can be used instead of the more expensive moist towelettes as a substitute for toilet paper.
3. Extracting thromboses, if present, can help relieve pain.
4. Rubber-band ligation, surgical excision, and chemical sclerosis are reserved for cases refractory to medical therapy.

ANAL FISSURE

What is it?	An abrasion or tear of the anal mucosa
What causes it?	A hard and/or large stool that tears or abrades the rectal mucosa
What are common symptoms?	Pain, especially with defecation Itching and blood spotting of the toilet paper may also be present.
What are common physical findings?	The tear or abrasion is identified when examining the rectum or on anoscopy. There is usually significant pain with digital rectal exam. No other tests are needed.
How are anal fissures treated?	Initial treatment is the same as with hemorrhoids, with emphasis on softening the stool. Defecation with initial urge to pass stool can be helpful in keeping stool size to a minimum, especially in patients who avoid defecation because of pain from the fissure. Be sure that moist wipes used to replace toilet paper do not contain alcohol, because the pain would be excruciating.

IRRITABLE BOWEL SYNDROME (IBS)

What is it?	A clinical syndrome characterized by alternating constipation and diarrhea with intermittent abdominal pain, bloating, and gas

What causes it?

It is thought that most symptoms are caused by autonomic hyperactivity, which leads to exaggerated gastrointestinal reflexes and peristalsis. The autonomic hyperactivity is usually a response to stress or anxiety.

What are common symptoms of IBS?

Passing of stool (often soft) 30 to 60 minutes after a meal is a frequent finding in addition to the symptoms noted above. The patient almost never has blood or mucus in the stool.

What are common physical findings of IBS?

The physical exam may show mildly hyperactive bowel sounds and mild, diffuse abdominal tenderness. However, the examination of the abdomen, rectum, and stool is usually completely normal.

What diagnostic tests are used?

If the clinical history and physical exam are strongly consistent with IBS, no tests are indicated. In situations where the diagnosis is unclear, IBS becomes a diagnosis of exclusion. Barium studies (e.g., barium enema with UGI and small-bowel follow-through or enteroclysis), colonoscopy, abdominal CT, CBC, ESR, stool for white cells, culture, and parasite evaluation are considered.

How is IBS treated?

1. Fiber supplements can make stool more consistent, so that the alternating constipation and diarrhea are less prominent.
2. Reassurance is helpful in reducing anxiety and, therefore, symptoms.
3. Anticholinergic agents can be used to decrease autonomic input but are usually reserved for the more difficult cases.

Helpful hints

1. Patient anxiety may force some testing even in cases where the diagnosis is clear. Limit the workup to the tests most applicable to the symptoms.
2. Use anticholinergics cautiously. Infections can be made worse and

prolonged by eliminating the ability of the gut to expel infecting organisms (i.e., impairing peristalsis). If the patient does not respond promptly, stop the drug and initiate evaluation promptly.

3. Initiate evaluation and therapy for significant anxiety simultaneously with any medical evaluation. Delaying behavioral evaluation and treatment until after medical evaluation can give the patient the impression that you think the symptoms are just "in their head." This impression is hard to dispel and can lead to difficulties in your future relationship.

PEPTIC ULCER DISEASE (PUD)

What is it?

Disruption of the mucosal surface of the stomach (gastric ulcer) or proximal duodenum (duodenal ulcer)

What are the two types of PUD?

1. Gastric ulcers
2. Duodenal ulcers

What causes gastric ulcers?

The most common cause is mucosal damage caused by NSAIDs. Other causes include *Helicobacter pylori* infection, excess acid secretion from a gastrin-secreting tumor, and ulcer formed by a gastric cancer.

What causes duodenal ulcers?

90% of duodenal ulcers are caused by *H. pylori* infection.

What are common symptoms of PUD?

Dull, aching epigastric abdominal pain is present in most (80%–90%) patients with PUD. It tends to improve with food or antacids and worsen with an empty stomach (e.g., between meals, at night). Nausea can occur but is less common. Vomiting is not usually present unless complications (e.g., active bleeding or obstruction caused by scar or tumor) are present. Melena can occur with significant bleeding.

Can duodenal and gastric ulcers be distinguished by symptoms?

No—symptoms are identical for both.

What are common physical findings of PUD?

Epigastric tenderness is the only common finding with PUD.

What diagnostic tests are used to demonstrate the location and severity of an ulcer?

UGI series and/or EGD

What diagnostic tests are used to detect *H. pylori*?

Biopsy of ulcer with histologic evaluation for *H. pylori* or CLO (Chlamydia-like organism) test, IgG and IgA antibody ELISA on serum, or a urea breath test. Both the breath test and CLO test use the presence of urea (a product of *H. pylori* metabolism) as an indirect indicator of *H. pylori* infection.

How is PUD treated?

1. Decrease gastric acid production.
2. Eliminate offending agents (NSAIDs).
3. Eradicate *H. pylori* when present.

What agents are used to decrease gastric acid?

Proton pump inhibitors (e.g., omeprazole) and H_2 receptor antagonists (e.g., ranitidine)

What agents are used to eradicate *H. pylori*?

A multidrug regimen that includes a proton pump inhibitor with 2–3 antibiotics for 2 weeks; effective antibiotics include bismuth, amoxicillin, metronidazole, and clarithromycin.

What agent has been effective in preventing ulcers caused by NSAIDs?

Misoprostol—it is used in patients at high risk of ulcers but who need NSAIDs for other problems (e.g., elderly patients or patients with previous ulcers)

What are potential complications of PUD?

Bleeding, which can be severe and life-threatening
Obstruction with anorexia and weight loss
Perforation of stomach or duodenum
Penetration of the ulcer into another organ (e.g., the pancreas)

What are the admission criteria?	1. Active bleeding 2. Blood loss requiring transfusion 3. Obstruction 4. Dehydration 5. Perforation or penetration (These criteria indicate potential medical emergencies and require urgent intervention. Surgical consult should be obtained early in the course of intervention. Coordination and cooperation between medical and surgical teams are essential.)
Helpful hints	1. Documented gastric ulcers without biopsy (seen on UGI or not biopsied during EGD) should have follow-up evaluation to document healing. Nonhealing gastric ulcers need biopsy to evaluate for cancer. 2. Coffee ground emesis or melena indicates significant bleeding and the patient requires further evaluation.

DIVERTICULAR DISEASE

What are the three common manifestations of diverticular disease?	1. Diverticulosis 2. Diverticulitis 3. Diverticular bleeding
What are diverticula?	Herniation(s) of mucosa and submucosa of the colon through the muscle layer, creating small pockets extending from the lumen of the colon
What is the term for the presence of diverticula?	Diverticulosis
How common is diverticulosis?	30% of persons over 60 years of age have diverticulosis.
What causes diverticulosis?	It is thought that diets low in fiber lead to smaller, harder stools that are more difficult to pass. This leads to increased intraluminal pressures required to pass the stool, which leads to herniation of the mucosa along the weaker points of the muscle wall.

What are common symptoms and signs of diverticulosis?

Two thirds of patients have no symptoms. The remaining one third usually have nonspecific symptoms, such as constipation or hemorrhoids. A small subset will have worse symptoms. Physical exam is not helpful for diagnosis.

What are complications of diverticulosis?

Diverticulitis and diverticular bleeding

What is diverticulitis?

An intra-abdominal infection with inflammation restricted to the pericolic area that results from rupture of a diverticulum

What are common signs and symptoms of diverticulitis?

Left lower abdominal pain, nausea, and vomiting are the most common symptoms. Low-grade fever with tenderness and palpable mass in the left lower quadrant of the abdomen are the classic physical findings.

What are complications of diverticulitis?

Abscess formation and perforation of the colon

What are the signs and symptoms of diverticular bleeding?

The patient usually has no symptoms but presents with bright red or maroon bleeding from the rectum. Abdominal exam is usually negative.

What are complications of diverticular bleeding?

Massive blood loss with hypotension, shock, and possible death

What diagnostic tests are used to diagnose diverticular diseases and complications?

1. Flexible sigmoidoscopy
2. Colonoscopy and barium enema can identify diverticula but are not indicated in asymptomatic patients; also, colonoscopy, barium enema, and CT can identify diverticulosis and abscess. Colonoscopy alone can identify active diverticular bleeding.
3. Plain abdominal radiographs can detect significant perforation and radiolabeled RBC studies, or mesenteric angiography can identify brisk active bleeding if colonoscopy is unsuccessful or contraindicated.

How are each of these entities treated?

Diverticulosis?

No specific therapy is indicated. Improving fiber content of the diet is thought to decrease long-term complications.

Diverticulitis?

Persons with mild symptoms can be treated as outpatients with oral antibiotics (e.g., metronidazole plus ciprofloxacin or trimethoprim/ sulfamethoxazole). Those with significant pain or vomiting need IV fluids and antibiotics (e.g., metronidazole plus a second- or third-generation cephalosporin). Significant abscess or perforation requires surgical intervention; surgical consult should be obtained if significant improvement does not occur in 2–3 days.

Diverticular bleeding?

Supportive care with fluid resuscitation and blood replacement are indicated while diagnostic studies are performed; 90% resolve spontaneously but surgical intervention is indicated if significant bleeding persists. Intra-arterial vasopressin is sometimes used if the bleeding source can be identified during angiography.

What are the admission criteria?

1. Significant recent or active rectal bleeding with or without hypotension and shock
2. Diverticulitis with significant pain, fever, nausea, vomiting, or dehydration—all of which would require IV therapy
3. Any patient that may require surgical consultation or intervention

Helpful hints

1. Diverticular bleeding is the most common cause of significant rectal bleeding. Cancers rarely cause frank bleeding.
2. Diverticula are more common in the distal portion of the colon; therefore, most symptoms and complications of diverticular disease are in the left lower quadrant.

INFLAMMATORY BOWEL DISEASE (IBD)

What are the two types of IBD?

Ulcerative colitis (UC) and Crohn's disease (regional enteritis)

What is UC?

An inflammatory process that involves only the mucosa of the colon

What is Crohn's disease?

An inflammatory process that involves the entire thickness of the gut. It can occur anywhere from the mouth to the anus, and it may be present in many discrete areas simultaneously.

How can UC and Crohn's disease of the colon be distinguished clinically?

Crohn's disease tends to have patchy lesions that are not contiguous with one another. These lesions are called *skip lesions,* because the inflammatory process does not involve, or skips, portions of mucosa. UC involves diffuse, contiguous areas of mucosa. Rectal abscess and fistulae occur with Crohn's disease; UC will have rectal inflammation only.

How can they be distinguished microscopically?

UC involves the mucosal layer only, whereas Crohn's disease is a transmural inflammatory process.

What are common signs and symptoms of IBD?

1. **Abdominal pain** and **loose stools with mucous or blood** are common to both types of IBD. UC tends to have left lower quadrant symptoms (pain and cramping) and bloody diarrhea, whereas Crohn's disease has more diffuse symptoms and insidious onset.
2. Physical exam shows **tenderness of the abdomen, fever,** and **weight loss.**
3. **Dehydration** may be present.
4. Rectal exam can reveal inflammation, fissures, abscess, and/or fistulae.

(The spectrum of disease is great. Patients can have minimal symptoms similar to IBS or fulminant symptoms with fever, weight loss, anemia, malnutrition, and intestinal obstruction.)

What diagnostic tests are used for IBD?

Colonoscopy, barium enema, and UGI with small bowel follow-through are used to identify involved areas of the GI tract. ESR identifies systemic evidence of inflammation. Hematocrit, vitamin B_{12}, and serum albumin reflect nutritional effects of the disease.

How are UC and Crohn's disease treated?

5-Aminosalicylic acid (5-ASA) derivatives, corticosteroids, and mercaptopurine are the main agents used. 5-ASA and corticosteroids can be given orally or as suppositories or enemas, depending on location and severity of disease; they are the first-line agents for both UC and Crohn's disease. Mercaptopurine is used for refractory Crohn's disease and has a high incidence (10%) of side effects. Advanced and/or severe disease with complications (e.g., obstruction, perforation, toxic megacolon) requires surgical therapy.

What are the admission criteria?

Evidence of significant dehydration, anemia, systemic toxicity (e.g., fever, vomiting, altered mental status), or acute blood loss. Complications, such as obstruction, toxic megacolon, and perforation, require admission with prompt supportive care and surgical evaluation.

Helpful hints

1. Obstruction occurs much more commonly with Crohn's disease since it can involve the small intestine.
2. A rectal abscess without an identified etiology should be considered a manifestation of Crohn's disease until proven otherwise.
3. Colonoscopy should be performed with great caution in patients with active UC, because the incidence of perforation by the scope is much higher than in a normal colon.
4. Twenty-five percent of patients with UC have extracolonic manifestations such as arthritis, erythema nodosum, and thromboembolic events.

5. UC increases the risk of colon cancer in proportion to the severity of disease. Careful screening is suggested. Previous recommendations for routine prophylactic colectomy are not supported by more recent data.

VIRAL HEPATITIS

What is it?

Diffuse hepatocellular inflammation of the liver secondary to viral infection

What are the types of viruses that cause viral hepatitis?

Hepatitis virus A (HAV)
Hepatitis virus B (HBV)
Hepatitis virus C (HCV)
Hepatitis virus D (HDV)
Non-A, non-B (NANB) hepatitis is thought to also be included in this classification.
(Other viruses that can cause hepatic inflammation, such as cytomegalovirus and Epstein-Barr virus, are not usually included in this classification.)

What are common signs and symptoms of viral hepatitis?

Nausea, vomiting, fatigue, weakness, anorexia, pruritus, and dark urine

What are common physical findings?

Jaundice, fever, hepatomegaly, and splenomegaly

What diagnostic tests are indicated?

Serum transaminases and bilirubin indicate the severity of the disease and are followed until resolution of the illness. The responsible virus is determined by serum antibody testing for the various agents.

Why is it important to determine the agent responsible for the hepatitis?

Public health concerns: Mode of transmission varies among the viruses and prevention measures for close contacts may be indicated.
Prognosis: HBV, HCV, and HDV can result in chronic carrier state or chronic infection with long-term risks of cirrhosis or hepatocellular cancer.

How is acute viral hepatitis treated?	Generally supportive measures, such as rest and antipyretics, are all that is indicated for the acute infection.
How is viral hepatitis transmitted?	HAV—fecal-oral route HBV, HVC, HDV, and NANB—body fluids (most commonly blood products and sexual contact) and maternal–fetal transmission
What public health measures help prevent viral transmission?	Good personal hygiene (especially handwashing and sewage treatment) and vaccination can prevent acquisition and spread of HAV. Testing blood donors, condom use, and single use of hypodermic needles can prevent transmission of HBV, HCV, and HDV. HBV can also be prevented by vaccination.
How are close contacts of persons with documented hepatitis treated?	Passive immunization with standard immune globulin or hepatitis B immune globulin (HBIG)
What are the admission criteria?	Admission is rarely needed. A dehydrated patient may need IV rehydration, and acute hepatic failure may require intensive care. If admitted, isolation measures for blood and other body fluids are required.
Helpful hints	1. Newborns of mothers with active HBV infection (acute or chronic) should be treated with HBIG and vaccination within 12 hours of birth. This prevention strategy is about 70% effective in prevention of transmission. 2. Patients recovering from acute hepatitis may return to work when transaminases return to normal even if jaundice has not resolved. 3. HDV can only cause infection in the presence of HBV.

9 ___

Common Genitourinary Problems

BENIGN PROSTATIC HYPERTROPHY (BPH)

What is it?

Diffuse, nonmalignant enlargement of the prostate gland that occurs in most men as they age

What causes it?

Unknown—but it is thought that the action of androgenic hormones on the prostate gland play a role in the development of hypertrophy

Is one portion of the prostate affected more than another?

Yes. The periurethral portion of the gland tends to enlarge more than the lateral lobes.

Do patients always have symptoms?

No. The patient is often asymptomatic.

What causes symptoms in the patients who have them?

The periurethral portion of the prostate gland becomes so enlarged that it compresses the urethra as it passes through the prostate, causing urinary tract symptoms.

What are common symptoms?

Difficulty initiating micturition
Dribbling of urine at the end of micturition
Urinary frequency (secondary to incomplete emptying of the bladder)
Decreased force and volume of the urine stream when voiding

What are common physical findings?

Digital rectal exam reveals a nontender, diffusely enlarged prostate.

What diagnostic tests are used?

Usually none. A history and physical exam consistent with BPH usually confirms the diagnosis. The American Urological Association Symptom Index may quantify symptom severity and document improvement with treatment. Serum prostate-specific antigen (PSA) test and/or transrectal ultrasound may be considered if cancer is suspected.

What is the medical treatment for BPH?

α-Adrenergic blockers (e.g., doxazosin) have been shown to improve both subjective symptoms and symptom scores. Androgenic inhibition with finasteride has also been helpful.

Which class of drugs is used as the first-line agent?

α-Adrenergic blockers

Why?

α-Blockers do not affect the PSA, and they have a prompt onset of action, whereas finasteride takes up to 6 months to show benefits and will decrease the PSA by about 50% (making it more difficult to interpret).

Do α-adrenergic blockers cause low blood pressure in nonhypertensive men?

No. They can be used safely to treat symptoms of BPH in patients with normal blood pressure.

What are surgical treatments for BPH?

Transurethral resection (with either sharp metal instrument or laser) and total prostatectomy have been used. Surgical options are usually reserved for those who fail medical therapy.

DYSFUNCTIONAL UTERINE BLEEDING (DUB)

What is it?

Uterine bleeding *not* secondary to menstruation

What causes it?

Menstrual cycle irregularities
Contraceptive agents
Ectopic pregnancy
Spontaneous abortion
Benign or malignant tumors

Why is the woman's age so important in evaluating DUB?

The risk of cancer increases as the woman ages.

What is the most common cause of DUB?

Anovulatory cycles

What is the mechanism of DUB with an anovulatory cycle?

Persistent estrogen effect promotes endometrial proliferation. Without the stabilizing effect of progesterone that normally comes from the corpus luteum following ovulation, the excessively proliferative endometrium tends to slough in an irregular and unpredictable pattern.

At what times during the reproductive years do women most commonly have anovulatory cycles?

At the beginning (at and near menarche) and end (perimenopausal) of their reproductive years

What physical exam findings indicate something other than anovulatory DUB?

Uterine or adnexal enlargement, irregularity, or tenderness could indicate bleeding secondary to threatened or spontaneous abortion, ectopic pregnancy, submucosal myoma, endometritis, endometrial hyperplasia, or cancer.
Physical exam should also reveal bleeding from areas other than the uterus (i.e., cervix, vagina).

What diagnostic tests are used to evaluate DUB?

The following test for anovulation, pregnancy, excessive blood loss, and tumors, respectively:
Basal body temperature chart
β-HCG test (urine or serum)
CBC
Endometrial biopsy; transvaginal ultrasound/hysteroscopy with or without dilatation and curettage (D&C)

What is the treatment for DUB?

Most women, especially younger women, respond to hormone therapy with some combination of estrogen and progestin. Persistent or recurrent bleeding may require D&C. Endometrial ablation or hysterectomy may be considered in women no longer desiring fertility.

What precautions must be taken with hormonal therapy in older women?
Because risk for endometrial cancer increases in frequency in peri- and postmenopausal women, perform endometrial biopsy before initiating any hormonal therapy for DUB. Postmenopausal women should have endometrial biopsy for all DUB.

What are the admission criteria?
1. Evidence of profound blood loss, such as low or decreasing hematocrit, orthostasis, or hypotension
2. Continued bleeding unresponsive to oral hormone therapy

Helpful hints
1. Endometrial biopsy is as reliable as D&C in detecting cancer. D&C should be reserved as a therapeutic tool (rather than for diagnosis) in most cases.
2. Women without DUB do not need endometrial biopsy before initiating hormone replacement therapy as a preventive measure.

DYSMENORRHEA

What is it?
Pelvic pain and cramping during menses

What causes it?
Prostaglandin release stimulates contraction of the smooth muscle of the uterus with menstruation.

What diagnostic tests are used?
Usually, tests are not indicated in a person with a typical history of symptoms with menses. Pelvic exam with cultures and/or ultrasound may be indicated in patients with atypical symptoms to evaluate for other potential causes of pelvic pain.

How is dysmenorrhea treated?
Prostaglandin inhibition with NSAIDs is the first line of therapy. Oral contraceptives are frequently used in patients unresponsive to NSAIDs.

What treatment is used if the patient is unresponsive to pharmacologic therapy?
Patients unresponsive to pharmacologic therapy may have a more complex disease, such as endometriosis.

Laparoscopy may be indicated as an additional diagnostic and therapeutic measure.

VAGINITIS

What is it?	Inflammation or irritation of the vagina
What is the most common cause?	Infection
What are the three types of vaginal infection?	1. Candidiasis 2. Trichomoniasis 3. Bacterial vaginosis
What are the common symptoms of vaginitis?	Burning, itching, and vaginal discharge
What are common physical findings with vaginitis?	Vaginal erythema, discharge, and odor
What physical findings indicate vaginal candidiasis?	Prominent erythema of the vulva and vagina with a thick, white discharge that resembles cottage cheese; usually no increase in vaginal odor with candidal infection
What physical findings indicate vaginal trichomoniasis?	Moderate erythema of the vagina with petechial lesions on the vaginal wall; the discharge is yellow, thin, bubbly, and malodorous
What physical findings indicate bacterial vaginosis?	No vaginal erythema; vaginal discharge is thin, malodorous, and a white-to-yellow color
What diagnostic tests are used to identify the etiology of vaginitis?	KOH and saline prep (see Chapter 2)
How is candidal vaginitis treated?	Topical antifungal vaginal creams (e.g., terconazole, miconazole) or oral fluconazole (a single 150-mg dose)
How is trichomonas vaginitis treated?	Oral metronidazole: a single, 2-g dose (i.e, four 500-mg tablets taken at once)

How is bacterial vaginosis treated?	Oral metronidazole: 1. 500 mg bid for 7 days is most effective (and is required if the patient is pregnant) 2. A one-time, 2-g dose can be used as an alternative regimen (only about 80% effective)
Which type of vaginitis is sexually transmitted?	Trichomonas vaginitis
Helpful hints	1. Recurrent candidal vaginitis may indicate systemic problems with the immune system (e.g., diabetes mellitus, HIV). 2. Bacterial vaginosis can cause premature labor and should be treated in all pregnant women.

URINARY TRACT INFECTION (UTI)

What is it?	Bacterial infection of the kidneys, renal collecting system, or urinary bladder
Are UTIs more common in men or women, and why?	Women—the urethra is much shorter and is subject to repetitive trauma during intercourse, which may introduce bacteria from the rectum and vagina into the urinary bladder.
What is the most common site of infection?	The urinary bladder
What is the term for infection of the urinary bladder?	Cystitis
What are common symptoms of cystitis?	Urinary urgency and frequency with dysuria
What are common physical findings with cystitis?	Mild-to-moderate suprapubic tenderness to palpation is the most common finding. The exam is usually otherwise normal.
What is the term for infection of the collecting system(s) and kidney(s)?	Pyelonephritis

What are common symptoms of pyelonephritis?	Fever, flank pain, nausea, and vomiting that is associated with and often preceded by urinary frequency, urgency, and dysuria.
What are common physical findings with pyelonephritis?	Fever and tenderness with percussion at the costovertebral angle of the back (CVA tenderness)
What tests are commonly used to diagnose UTI?	Urinalysis (dip and microscopic examination of a spun specimen; see Chapter 2) Urine culture
What microscopic findings are common in UTI?	WBCs ($> 5/HPF$) RBCs Bacteria
What microscopic finding indicates pyelonephritis?	WBC casts
Is a urine culture indicated for every UTI?	No. Uncomplicated cystitis can usually be treated empirically, in which urine culture is reserved if treatment is unsuccessful.
How are UTIs treated?	With antibiotics that cover the gram-negative coliform bacteria, which most frequently causes UTIs
What are the most commonly used first-line agents?	Trimethoprim/sulfamethoxazole Amoxicillin Macrodantin
What are the most commonly used second-line agents?	Quinolones Cephalosporins Aminoglycosides
What is the duration of therapy?	With the exception of uncomplicated cystitis, treatment is 7–14 days, depending on severity of infection.
What is uncomplicated cystitis?	It is cystitis in an otherwise healthy, sexually active woman. It excludes men and children with a UTI as well as women with: 1. Signs and symptoms of pyelonephritis 2. Other medical problems

3. History of urinary tract surgery
4. Instrumentation or malformation
5. Failed treatment of cystitis
6. Excessively frequent cystitis (> 2–3 episodes yearly)
7. Pregnancy

How is uncomplicated cystitis treated?

Trimethoprim/sulfamethoxazole or amoxicillin for 3 days

What are additional concerns if a man or child has a UTI?

Because there are no predisposing factors for UTI, the incidence of structural abnormality or vessiculoureteral (VU) reflux is greatly increased. Further evaluation with intravenous pyelogram (IVP), ultrasound, and/or voiding cystourethrogram is usually indicated.

What are the admission criteria?

1. Nausea and/or vomiting that preclude the patient taking oral antibiotics
2. High fever with hypotension and dehydration, indicating possibility of sepsis
3. Children < 1 year of age
4. All pregnant women with evidence of pyelonephritis
5. Elderly or institutionalized patients with other medical problems (at increased risk for sepsis)

Helpful hints

1. Sexually active women with frequent UTIs can decrease frequency if they void after intercourse.
2. Cystitis can cause significant hematuria, but the urine should be reevaluated after treatment is completed to ensure that there is no residual hematuria. Hematuria after treatment and resolution of symptoms should initiate evaluation for calculi, tumors, and/or renal disease.
3. Any patient with an indwelling Foley catheter is at increased risk of acquiring resistant organisms, and treatment with broader spectrum agent should be initiated pending culture.

RENAL CALCULI

What are they?	Solid precipitates (stones) that occur in the renal collecting system
What are the most common components of the calculi?	Calcium oxalate and urate
What causes calculi?	Excessive concentrations of calcium or uric acid cause solid precipitates to form in the collecting system.
What are common symptoms of renal calculi?	Intermittent (colicky) severe flank pain that is associated with nausea and vomiting; patients frequently have a past history of calculi
What are common physical findings with renal calculi?	Diaphoresis and pallor are frequently found. The patient will have difficulty sitting or lying still because of the severe pain. Otherwise, the exam is usually unremarkable.
What diagnostic tests are used?	Urinalysis (dip and microscopy) Radiographs of kidneys and upper bladder (KUB) IVP and/or renal ultrasound
What is usually found on urinalysis?	Isolated hematuria with 5 or more RBCs per HPF
What is the gold standard radiologic test?	IVP—it locates the position of the stone and identifies obstruction. KUB and ultrasound can sometimes identify the stone, and ultrasound can identify significant obstruction.
How are renal calculi treated?	1. Initially, analgesics are used for pain control and the urine is strained to recover the stone. 2. If the stone doesn't pass within 5–10 days or if complications (e.g., persistent pain, obstruction, infection) occur, urologic referral is indicated; the stone is recovered via basket extraction, ureteroscopy, and/or lithotripsy.

How are they prevented?

Calcium stones—patients are instructed to maintain a low calcium diet and can be given medication to improve calcium solubility in the urine

Urate stones—by administering agents that decrease the production of uric acid (e.g., allopurinol)

What are the admission criteria?

1. Nausea and vomiting that preclude taking oral analgesics or cause dehydration
2. Evidence of obstruction with infection requires parenteral antibiotics and urologic referral.

Helpful hints

1. Pain is associated with movement of the stone. Obstruction occurs without pain because the stone has stopped moving.
2. Obstruction by stones can lead to infection. Persons with symptoms of pyelonephritis and a history of renal calculi need careful evaluation.

IMPOTENCE

What is it?

A type of sexual dysfunction in which the patient is unable to initiate or maintain an erection. Although most men have an isolated episode of erectile dysfunction at some time, impotence is usually reserved for recurrent or persistent problems.

What is the most common cause?

Psychological factors (e.g., anxiety, guilt, depression)

What are other common causes?

Drugs, including alcohol
Vascular disease
Diabetes mellitus
Inadequate testosterone production

What are common symptoms?

Primarily, the symptom is erectile dysfunction.

How should the patient be evaluated?

Past medical history: should be reviewed to identify medications and problems that may cause impotence.

Patient's feelings: Should be reviewed regarding intimacy, performance, guilt, and the relationship with present partner or partners should be explored to identify potential psychological factors that may influence the problem.

Overall stress level: Gauge the stress level in the patient's life, because stressors unrelated to sexuality and/or relationships may affect sexual performance.

What key factor in the patient's history can identify most cases of impotence due to psychological factors?

Nocturnal tumescence (i.e., nighttime erections). Most men with psychologic impotence continue to have erections in their sleep and when they awake early in the morning. Nocturnal tumescence indicates that the hormonal-neuro-vascular systems are intact and functioning.

What are common physical findings?

Most of the time, the physical exam is normal. Testicular atrophy, prostate mass, hypertension, or abnormal vascular or neurologic exams may indicate potential organic causes.

What diagnostic tests are used?

Nocturnal tumescence tests
Serum testosterone
Fasting blood glucose (to diagnose occult diabetes)

What is the stamp test, and how is it performed?

It is a test of nocturnal tumescence. Several stamps from a roll are placed snugly around the flaccid penis at bedtime (glue side away from the penis with a one-stamp overlap). The overlapping stamps are glued together, using the glue on the stamp. Nocturnal tumescence is confirmed if the ring of stamps is broken in the morning.

How is impotence treated?

1. Counseling with reassurance can help most patients with psychological impotence.
2. Maximizing therapy for medical conditions contributing to impotence

(e.g., diabetes mellitus, vascular disease) can limit progression. Treatment regimens that include drugs that cause impotence can be altered.

3. Testosterone-deficient patients can receive replacement therapy. Desipramine, yohimbine, or topical nitrates can help some patients.

4. Intracorporeal injections of papaverine, phentolamine, or prostaglandin E_1 are effective but must be injected each time the patient desires an erection.

5. External vacuum devices and penile implants are also used.

Helpful hints

1. Impotence is anxiety producing. Psychosocial support is necessary regardless of the etiology of the problem. The patient may need counseling even if an organic cause is identified.

2. Consider urologic referral early in the process if the etiology cannot readily be identified.

SEXUALLY TRANSMITTED DISEASES (STDs)

What are they?

A group of infectious diseases that are transmitted by exposure to the body fluids of an infected person during any type of sexual activity.

Is this the only way these agents can be transmitted?

No. Some STDs (e.g., hepatitis B and HIV) can be transmitted through blood products and/or from mother to fetus during pregnancy (i.e., vertical transmission).

What are common STDs?

Gonorrhea
Syphilis
Chlamydia
Ureaplasma
Genital herpes simplex virus (HSV)
Human papillomavirus (HPV)
HIV

Hepatitis B virus
Trichomonas

What are common clinical syndromes caused by STDs?

Urethritis
Vaginitis
Cervicitis
Genital lesions (single or multiple; painless or painful)
Pelvic inflammatory disease (PID)
Systemic viremia (e.g., fever, chills, weakness, nausea)
AIDS
Genital tract dysplasia
Infertility

How can STDs be prevented?

The only method that is 100% effective is abstinence. Maintaining a mutually monogamous sexual relationship with a person without STDs can also be effective if past exposures are limited and testing is accurate. Use of latex condoms can prevent transmission of most (but not all) STDs, if used properly.

GONORRHEA

What two common clinical syndromes does it cause?

Urethritis and cervicitis

What diagnostic tests are used?

Culture or DNA probe of urethra or cervix

How is it treated?

Antibiotics—there are many effective regimens, but the treatment of choice is ceftriaxone (250 mg IM)

What are complications of untreated gonorrhea?

In women—PID
In men—epididymitis
(Both can lead to scarring and infertility)
Rarely, septic arthritis can occur secondary to gonorrhea.

What special considerations exist for pregnant patients?

Gonorrhea can be transmitted to the infant as it passes through the birth canal, resulting in purulent conjunctivitis. All infants have antibiotic ointment applied to the eyes shortly after birth to prevent this.

CHLAMYDIA/UREAPLASMA

What common clinical syndromes do they cause?

Urethritis and cervicitis

What diagnostic tests are used?

DNA probe or tissue culture can test for chlamydia. No diagnostic tests are available for clinical use to detect ureaplasma.

What are the first-line agents used to treat chlamydia/ureaplasma?

Doxycycline: 100 mg bid for 10 days *or* Azithromycin: a single 1-g dose

What are other effective agents?

Erythromycin, amoxicillin, tetracycline, and selected quinolones

What are complications of untreated chlamydia/ureaplasma?

PID (in women) and epididymitis (in men), which can lead to scarring and infertility

What are the contraindications for pregnant patients?

Doxycycline (and other tetracycline antibiotics) and quinolones

HSV

What common clinical syndrome does it cause?

Painful genital ulcers, which are about 2–4 mm in diameter and have an erythematous base; because dormant virus exists in the dorsal root ganglia after resolution of the primary infection, recurrent episodes from reactivation of the virus are common

What diagnostic tests are used?

Viral culture of active lesions

How is it treated?

Acyclovir and famciclovir decrease the duration of lesions and viral shedding. They do not eliminate the virus. Persons with frequent recurrences can be treated prophylactically to decrease the number of recurrences.

What are complications of HSV?	Cancer of the penis, vulva, vagina, and cervix are thought to be associated with HSV infection. Because recurrences are unpredictable and the virus is not curable, a great deal of stress associated with sexual activity and relationships can be present. A high incidence of asymptomatic viral shedding complicates the social issues even further.
What special considerations exist for pregnant patients?	Transmission of HSV to the baby from active lesions on the cervix as the baby passes through the birth canal, which can result in a systemic HSV infection in the newborn with a potentially devastating outcome. This is most likely if the maternal HSV infection is a primary infection (not a recurrence). Traditionally, a C-section is performed if the mother has active lesions on the cervix when she goes into labor, but recent data indicate that infant outcomes are not improved by this strategy. Acyclovir given throughout the third trimester may help decrease the rate of active lesions at the onset of labor and, therefore, decrease the C-section rate.

HPV

What common clinical syndrome does it cause?	Genital warts
What diagnostic tests are used?	Biopsy or viral culture with viral typing can be used but the diagnosis is usually made clinically.
How is it treated?	Cryotherapy, tri- or bichloracetic acid, podophyllin, or a laser can be used to destroy the lesions.
What are complications of HPV?	Dysplasia and cancer of the vulva, vagina, cervix, and penis are associated with HPV infection.
How is the epidemiology of HPV different from other STDs?	HPV transmission is not prevented by the use of condoms.

What special considerations exist for pregnant patients?

HPV can be transmitted to the baby as it passes through the birth canal with variable clinical outcomes, most of which are not severe. However, warts can occur in the trachea (with compromise of airway) of an exposed infant.

HIV

What common clinical syndromes does it cause?

Initial infection can cause a wide spectrum of clinical symptoms from a mild, flu-like illness to severe symptoms with hepatitis, meningitis, and dehydration. After recovery from the initial infection, there is a period in which the patient has no symptoms but can transmit the virus. AIDS is the final stage of HIV infection, in which the patient's CD4 counts drop below 500, and the patient has a series of opportunistic infections or malignancies that ultimately lead to death.

What diagnostic tests are used?

Initial screening is done by an enzyme-linked immunoassay (ELISA) test for antibodies to HIV. A positive ELISA is confirmed by a Western Blot test for HIV antibodies. The Western Blot is much more specific but also more expensive; thus it is reserved for confirming positive initial screening ELISAs. Polymerase chain reaction testing for HIV is presently used to identify and quantitate viral load and sensitivity to therapy. CD4 counts follow the effects of the virus on susceptible cells and can help predict the onset of opportunistic infections (AIDS).

How is HIV treated?

Antiretroviral therapy is initiated as soon as the patient is identified as HIV positive. Multiple drug regimens are used. Antiretroviral drugs are being developed and released very rapidly and treatment recommendations are changing along with these developments. Generally, multiple agents are used simultaneously to prevent viral replication; this has been shown to slow the progression of disease (as documented by decreased viral load and increased CD4 counts).

What are complications of HIV infection?

AIDS and death are the most obvious. Anxiety, guilt, relationship difficulties, and financial difficulties (antiretroviral therapy is very expensive) are a few examples of the multitude of psychosocial complications of HIV.

What special considerations exist for pregnant patients?

Vertical transmission of HIV to the fetus occurs in about 30% of pregnancies. This can be reduced to about 10% transmission if the mother is treated with AZT during the third trimester and if the infant is treated after birth. It is imperative to identify all HIV-positive women in pregnancy to achieve the benefit of treatment.

HEPATITIS B

What common clinical syndromes does it cause?

Acute and chronic hepatitis

What diagnostic tests are used?

Tests for viral antigens and antibodies to viral antigens are used to identify acute and chronic infection as well as identify the risk of transmission by chronic carriers of the virus.

How is it treated?

There is no treatment (other than supportive care) for patients with acute hepatitis. The best strategy is prevention.

How is hepatitis B prevented?

Hepatitis B vaccine is recommended for all ages. Postexposure treatment with hepatitis B immune globulin (HBIG) is recommended for unimmunized persons immediately after an exposure that places them at risk for infection (e.g., health care workers with a needle stick accident).

What are complications of hepatitis B infection?

Chronic active hepatitis occurs in varying rates (from 10% of adults to up to 50% of infants) following acute infection, and it eventually leads to cirrhosis and/or hepatocellular carcinoma (the time course is variable and may be prolonged). A chronic carrier state without chronic hepatitis can exist. These persons are at higher risk of hepatocellular carcinoma but not cirrhosis. They can transmit the virus.

What special considerations exist for pregnant patients?

Mothers with chronic hepatitis or who are chronic carriers can transmit the virus to the baby during birth. Acute infection in the newborn can be prevented by a combination of HBIG and vaccine if administered promptly after birth. Therefore, it is recommended that all pregnant women be tested for evidence of past hepatitis B early in pregnancy so that the newborn can be promptly treated.

TRICHOMONAS

What common clinical syndrome does it cause?

Vaginitis

What diagnostic test is used?

Saline prep (see Chapter 2)

How is it treated?

Metronidazole: a single 2-g dose (four 500-mg tablets taken at once)

What are complications of trichomonas vaginitis?

Cystitis

What special considerations exist for pregnant patients?

No specific concerns other than the possibility of other STDs being present

Helpful hints

1. Because many viral STDs have similar initials (e.g., HSV, HPV, HIV), it is best to use the full name of the virus, rather than the initials, when discussing the presence of an

infection by these agents. This will prevent undue anxiety and confusion that can occur if the patient hears *HIV* instead of *HPV*.

2. If one STD is present, test for other common STDs.

10   Common Hematologic Problems

ANEMIA

What are the defining laboratory features in men and women?	Women: Hemoglobin < 12 g/dl or hematocrit < 38% Men: Hemoglobin < 13.5 g/dl or hematocrit < 40% (There are age-specific indices for pediatric populations.)
What accounts for the difference in normal ranges between men and women?	Testosterone-induced hematopoiesis

TYPES OF ANEMIA

What is the most common cause of anemia?	Iron deficiency (by far the most common worldwide)
What are other clinically important types of anemia?	Anemia of chronic disease Sideroblastic anemia Megaloblastic anemia *More rare:* Anemias caused by liver or renal failure, lead poisoning, and endocrinopathies
What are the three most common causes of iron deficiency?	1. Blood loss 2. Malabsorption (e.g., because of gastrectomy, achlorhydria, celiac disease) 3. Decreased intake or increased utilization (as occurs in pregnancy or, rarely, because of dietary deficiencies)
What are the two major causes of chronic blood loss causing iron deficiency anemia?	1. Menstruation 2. GI disorders, especially in men and postmenopausal women

What are the major causes of GI blood loss?
Gastritis, peptic ulcer disease, varices, inflammatory bowel disease, arteriovenous malformations, diverticula, parasites

What are four causes of anemia of chronic disease?
1. Acute or chronic infections
2. Rheumatoid disease
3. Malignancy
4. Decubitus ulcer

What are sideroblastic anemias?
A heterogeneous group of disorders characterized by ineffective erythropoiesis, which result in two circulating populations of red cells—normal and microcytic/hypochromic. Ringed sideroblasts are seen on bone marrow examination (hence the name).

What causes megaloblastic anemia?
A defect in DNA synthesis with normal RNA and protein synthesis leads to large red cells (i.e., elevated mean corpuscular volume; MCV). The main cause of this defect is deficiency of cobalamin (vitamin B_{12}) and/or folate. It is important to determine which is deficient, because although folate administration corrects the megaloblastosis of either cause, it may worsen the neuropsychopathology associated with cobalamin deficiency.

CLINICAL COURSE

See Figure 10–1 and Tables 10–1 and 10–2 for diagnostic approaches for anemia.

What are important historical factors in patients with anemia?
Menstrual history, dietary history, alcohol consumption, chronic medical problems, medication use, family history of anemia, stool color and pattern, heavy metal exposure (especially lead), recent infection

What are signs and symptoms of anemia?
Pica (the urge to eat unusual substances such as dirt), fatigue, decreasing exercise performance, pallor of mucous membranes and conjunctiva

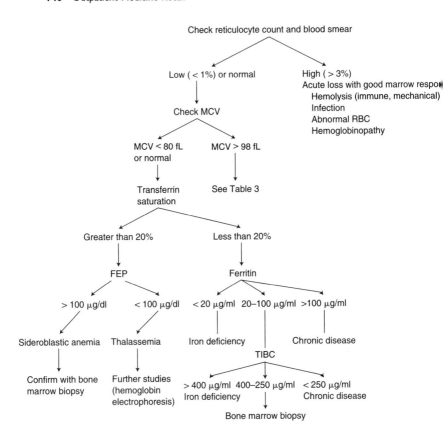

Table 10-1. Microcytic Anemia Tests

	Serum Iron (ng/ml)	TIBC (µg/ml)	Transferrin Saturation (%)	Serum Ferritin (ng/ml)	FEP (nM/g hgb)
Normal	60–100	250–400	30–60	20–100	< 100
Iron deficiency	< 60	> 400	< 20	< 20	> 100
Chronic disease	< 60	< 250	< 20	> 100	> 100
Sideroblastic anemia	> 100	250–400	> 60	20–100	> 100

FEP = free erythrocyte protoprophyrin; *TIBC* = total iron-binding capacity.

Table 10-2. Macrocytic Anemia Tests

	Serum B_{12}	Serum Folate	RBC Folate	Methylmalonic Acid	Homo-cysteine
Vitamin B_{12} deficiency	Low	High–normal	Low–normal	High	High
Folate deficiency	Normal	Low	Low	Normal	High
Vitamin B_{12} *and* folate deficiency	Low	Low	Low	°°°	°°°

RBC = red blood cell

What diagnostic tests are used to determine the cause of anemia?	CBC with red cell indices [mean corpuscular volume (MCV), mean corpuscular hemoglobin concentration (MCHC), red blood cell distribution width index (RDW)]
	Reticulocyte count
	Red cell morphology (examination of peripheral smear)
	Serum iron
	Ferritin, total iron-binding capacity (TIBC)
	Lead
	Hemoglobin electrophoresis
	Free erythrocyte protoporphyrin (FEP)
	Bone marrow biopsy
How is anemia treated?	The most effective treatment is to identify the underlying cause and treating it (e.g., replacing iron in patients with iron deficiency anemia).
	Transfusion temporarily helps patients with critically low hematocrits.
	Erythropoietin is given to patients with anemia of chronic disease who have low endogenous production or erythropoietin (e.g., those with chronic renal failure).
What are the admission criteria for a patient with anemia?	Evidence of ongoing acute blood loss (e.g., acute GI bleed)
	Profound anemia impairing oxygen delivery to critical organs (e.g., heart, brain, kidneys), especially if preexisting impairment of these organs exists
	Hypotension with hemodynamic compromise

Helpful hints	1. Reticulocyte count: immature red blood cells

Corrected reticulocyte count
$$= \frac{\text{absolute count} \times \text{patient's hematocrit}}{45\%}$$

2. Transferrin: iron transport molecule. Transferrin varies inversely with iron stores. It is falsely elevated by pregnancy or oral contraceptives. Acute stressors can falsely lower this value.
3. TIBC: measures the amount of transferrin in circulation
4. Transferrin saturation:[(serum iron / TIBC) $\times$ 100].
5. Ferritin: iron storage protein. Ferritin is an acute-phase reactant—i.e., during acute or chronic inflammatory disorders, liver/kidney disease, or malignancy, ferritin may be elevated disproportionately to iron stores. This increase may be seen as a potential confounding factor of these conditions. However, some iron stores must be present to allow this disproportionate elevation. Therefore, a ferritin in the upper range of normal or an elevated ferritin rules out iron deficiency anemia.
6. FEP: precursor of heme, elevated in disorders of heme synthesis (i.e., iron deficiency, sideroblastic anemia, lead poisoning)

LYMPHADENOPATHY

What is it?	Enlarged, sometimes painful lymph nodes
What are the causes of lymphadenopathy?	Infection—bacterial, viral, mycotic, mycobacterial, parasitic Immunologic—serum sickness, sarcoidosis, rheumatic disease, drug reaction Malignant—hematologic versus nonhematologic Miscellaneous—endocrinopathies, lipidoses

What is the risk of malignancy in a patient with lymphadenopathy?	The risk for a malignant cause increases with the patient's age: Patient's age < 30 years—80% of lymphadenopathy is benign Patient's age > 50 years—40% of lymphadenopathy is benign
What are four important historical factors?	1. Localized versus generalized (focal or systemic etiology) 2. Time to develop (nodes greater than 4–6 weeks worrisome) 3. Associated symptoms (e.g., viral syndrome preceding cervical adenopathy) 4. Location (supraclavicular more worrisome than cervical)

What are three important features of enlarged lymph nodes?	1. Tenderness (suggests infectious cause)
	2. Consistency
	  ° Warm, fluctuant, with erythema—infectious
	  ° Hard, fixed under skin—carcinoma (metaplastic)
	  ° Firm, rubbery—lymphoma
	3. Size—greater than $2\frac{1}{4}$ cm worrisome for neoplasia

What diagnostic tests are commonly used in patients with lymphadenopathy?	CBC with differential PPD (tuberculin skin test) Serum antibody test for HIV Fine-needle aspiration or excision for pathologic evaluation
Helpful hints	Can observe (+/− antibiotics) if the onset is new, the local cause is identified, and the malignancy risk is low If malignancy risk is (1) high or (2) low, but with persistent enlarged nodes, then fine-needle aspiration or excisional biopsy is necessary.

SICKLE CELL DISEASE

What is it?	Abnormal hemoglobin that polymerizes in the deoxygenated state and damages the erythrocyte cell membrane

What causes it?
A single mutation from GAG to GUG at the sixth amino acid of the beta chain of the globin molecule, which changes glutamine to valine

What ethnic groups carry this gene?
It is most commonly found in the African-American population, although it is also found in other groups of Mediterranean descent.

What is the inheritance pattern for the sickle cell gene?
Autosomal recessive

What percent of African Americans are carriers?
8%

Are carriers affected?
They have no significant problems, and they do not need activity restrictions. However, there are implications for family planning.

What is the advantage (darwinian) to carriers of this gene?
Heterozygote carriers are more resistant to malaria. Therefore, in areas of endemic infestation with malaria, carriers have a selective advantage.

What are the acute clinical syndromes commonly seen in sickle cell patients?
Painful crises: They affect over 50% of patients and can have multiple locations (often back and thighs).
Acute chest syndrome: It affects 10%–20% of adults with pain and chest radiograph infiltrate. It may be difficult to differentiate from pneumonia and has high mortality.
Priapism: It affects 10%–40% of men and can lead to impotence.
Sepsis and/or osteomyelitis

What are the chronic clinical syndromes commonly seen in sickle cell patients?
Aseptic bone necrosis, especially of the hips and shoulders; affects 10%–25% of adult patients
Functional asplenia, which affects greater than 90% of individuals (often by age 10) and predisposes them to sepsis caused by encapsulated organisms (e.g., *Streptococcus pneumoniae, Haemophilus influenzae*)

Gallstones
Nephropathy, which is a late
   complication

What is the major cause of   Infection
death in a patient with
sickle cell disease?

What problems may sickle   10%–20% spontaneous abortion rate;
cell disease cause with   gene transmission
pregnancy?

What preventive   Immunizations (pneumovax, *H.*
treatments are used in   *influenzae*)
patients with sickle cell   Nutrition (folic acid supplements for
disease?   new red cell production)
                       Prophylactic penicillin (starting at 3–4
                          months of age)

What treatments are used   IV fluids
in patients with sickle cell   Pain medication (e.g., NSAIDS,
disease who have acute   narcotics, patient-controlled analgesia)
symptoms?   Aggressive search for infection (and low
                          threshold for antibiotics)
                       Transfusion if hematocrit decreases
                          severely
                       Supplemental oxygen
                       Hydroxyurea

What are the admission   All of the acute complications usually
criteria?   require hospital admission for treatment.

How does hydroxyurea   Hydroxyurea causes increased
therapy assist patients with   production of fetal hemoglobin in red
sickle cell disease?   blood cells. Fetal hemoglobin lacks the
                       beta chain so the red blood cell will not
                       sickle.

11

Common Musculoskeletal Problems

BACK PAIN

What is it?	The subjective feeling of pain in or around the axial skeleton
How common is it?	Up to 80% of adults have at least one episode of low back pain in their lives. Back pain is one of the leading causes of time lost from work and long-term disability leave from work.
What causes it?	Trauma or acute strain of muscles or tendons Fractures Overuse injuries Mechanical impingement syndromes Osteoporosis Autoimmune disease (e.g., ankylosing spondylitis) Infection Tumors Chronic pain syndromes of unclear etiology (e.g., chronic fatigue syndrome or fibromyalgia syndrome)
What are common modulators of back pain?	Stress, anxiety, and depression often exacerbate back pain.
What are important factors to address when taking a history in a patient with back pain?	Exact mechanism of injury (if trauma precipitated pain) Duration and location of pain Mitigating factors (what makes it worse or better) Presence of weakness or changes in sensation

Athletic participation (competitive and
recreational)
Risk factors for osteoporosis
Continence of urine or feces (autonomic
nerve dysfunction)
Family history of back problems or
arthritis
General level of stress in the patient's
life

**What are the common
symptoms associated with
back pain?**

Stiffness and loss of range of motion
Worsening of pain with movement
Radiation of pain to other areas
Neurologic symptoms such as numbness
or tingling along a dermatome

**Name the important
components of the physical
examination in patients
with back pain.**

Location of tender areas
Testing the range of motion in all
directions (flexion, extension, rotation,
and sideways bending)
Testing for neurologic deficits (motor,
sensory, deep tendon reflexes)
Checking the effect on the pain of
straight leg raises (full extension of the
knee with flexion of the hip to 90)

**What are the most
common radiologic tests
used to evaluate back
pain?**

Plain radiography
Computed tomography (CT)
Magnetic resonance imaging (MRI)
Myelography (with or without CT)
Radionuclide bone scan

**What other tests are
considered in some
patients?**

CBC
Erythrocyte sedimentation rate (ESR)
Rheumatoid factor (RF)
Anti-nuclear antibody (ANA)
Nerve conduction studies

**What medications are used
to treat back pain?**

- Acetaminophen and NSAIDs are the
first-line analgesics used in most cases
of back pain.
- Narcotic analgesics and muscle
relaxants are used as second-line
agents.
- Pain pathway modulators (tricyclic
antidepressants [TCAs] and antiepileptic agents [carbamazepine or
gabapentin]) can be helpful with

chronic pain (pain of longer than 6 weeks' duration).

What are some other recommendations for back pain?

Allow patients to be as active as they can tolerate. Avoid bed rest. Range of motion exercises and physical therapy for strengthening may help some patients. Electronic nerve stimulation, heat, or ice may help control pain as well. Injection of trigger points or irritated nerve roots with a local anesthetic and corticosteroids can be helpful. Chiropractic manipulation has been shown to be beneficial in the treatment of chronic back pain.

What role does surgery have in the treatment of back pain?

Patients with mechanical impingement syndromes can benefit from surgical decompression.

What are the two most common mechanical impingement syndromes?

1. Herniated nucleus pulposis (HNP) of an intervertebral disc
2. Spinal canal stenosis

Is surgery always indicated for HNP?

No. Conservative therapy is indicated initially. If the patient does not respond to analgesia and physical therapy, surgery can be considered.

Why?

Studies have shown that, while short-term symptoms (1 year) are improved by surgical intervention, long-term symptoms (5 years) are not improved. Therefore, the clinical course and response to therapy must be closely monitored in each patient with HNP. The practitioner should discuss the risks and benefits of surgical intervention with patients who do not respond to conservative therapy.

How can back pain be prevented?

Using proper lifting techniques
Ergonomic design of work stations to minimize repetitive movements that stress the muscles and tendons of the back

Appropriate stretching before and after athletic participation (competitive and recreational)

Calcium, vitamin D, and hormone replacement therapy in post-menopausal women

Helpful hints

1. Radiographs of the involved region of the spine should be carefully considered before referral for physical therapy. Radiographs will usually exclude bone pathology that could make physical therapy dangerous.
2. Alternative therapies such as acupuncture can be helpful in patients who don't respond to other treatment.
3. 30% of asymptomatic persons will have an abnormal intervertebral disc on MRI. Therefore, HNP on MRI does not necessarily correlate with etiology of pain.
4. Eighty-five percent of patients with acute back pain will improve within 6 weeks.

What are the admission criteria?

Unrelenting, incapacitating pain that precludes a person from self-care will rarely prompt hospital admission. An unstable fracture of a vertebra and spinal cord compression by tumors are medical emergencies that require hospital admission and prompt specialty consultation and intervention.

OSTEOPOROSIS

What is it?

Loss of bone mineralization and density without other abnormalities in bone architecture

What is the most common cause?

Lack of estrogen in women after menopause (both natural and surgical)

What are risk factors?

Female sex
Lean body mass (i.e., thinness)
Tobacco use

Family history
Early menopause
European or Asian ancestry

What are common signs and symptoms of osteoporosis?

Early in the course of the process there are none. Later, the patient may have fractures with minor trauma, or progressive kyphosis with loss of stature.

What tests are used to diagnose osteoporosis?

Plain radiographs—show decreased mineralization; qualitative and somewhat subjective test
Bone density studies—direct measurement that gives a quantitative result which can be used to calculate relative risk of fracture in the bones studied

How is bone density measured?

Quantitative CT scan or absorptiometry

What is the goal of prevention and treatment of osteoporosis?

The goal is reduction in the number of fractures in patients with the disease. Prevention and treatment strategies that increase density readings but do not affect fracture rates should be viewed with skepticism.

How is osteoporosis prevented?

Smoking cessation
Weight-bearing exercise
Calcium (1500 mg/day) and vitamin D (400 IU/day) supplementation
Estrogen replacement therapy (ERT)

When should prevention be initiated?

Weight-bearing exercise and calcium/vitamin D supplementation should begin years before menopause is expected. ERT should begin at menopause.

Why is it important to begin ERT at menopause?

ERT preserves bone mineralization; it does not increase mineralization. The greatest loss of bone mass is in the first decade after menopause. So, in order for ERT to be most effective, it should be initiated early. This allows for the greatest preservation of bone mass possible.

What are some of the possible complications of ERT?	Resumption of vaginal bleeding (if the cyclical method is used) Increased risk of endometrial carcinoma (this risk is eliminated if progesterone is used with estrogen) Possible increased risk of breast cancer (conflicting data: some studies show no increased risk while other studies have shown some increased risk)
What agents are used to treat osteoporosis?	Biphosphonates (alendronate, etidronate) Calcitonin nasal spray
Helpful hints	1. ERT's greatest benefit is the reduction in CAD in women taking ERT. This benefit greatly exceeds any risk of endometrial or breast neoplasms. 2. Bone density is not indicated as a screening test except in women with very high risk. There is no evidence that using this as a screening test decreases fracture rates.

JOINT EFFUSION

What is it?	The collection of an abnormal amount or abnormal type of fluid (i.e., fluids other than synovial fluid) within the capsule of a joint
What causes it?	Trauma (acute and chronic) Infection Inflammation Precipitation of crystals Autoimmune processes
What are common signs and symptoms?	Pain Stiffness Limited range of motion Warmth and erythema of the overlying skin Tenderness and swelling or "fullness" of the joint to palpation Effusion secondary to a traumatic injury (can also be associated with laxity or disruption of the supporting ligaments)

What diagnostic tests are frequently used to evaluate joint effusions?

Plain radiographs are frequently used to evaluate for evidence of chronic arthritis or fracture. Joint aspiration with analysis of synovial fluid can be very helpful in diagnosis (for technique, see Chapter 2); synovial fluid analysis includes checking for the presence or absence of blood (hemarthrosis), white blood cell count (WBC), culture, glucose level, evaluation for crystals, and viscosity testing. Complete blood count (CBC), erythrocyte sedimentation rate, uric acid level, rheumatoid factor, and antinuclear antibody tests are often used in evaluating effusions not associated with trauma.

How are they treated?

Large effusions (especially in the larger joints) are very uncomfortable; aspiration of the majority of fluid in the joint can help relieve pain. However, treatment of the underlying process that caused the effusion is essential to long-term treatment success. Without this, the effusion will re-accumulate in a short period of time after aspiration.

Helpful hints

1. Effusion secondary to acute infection in the joint (septic arthritis) is a surgical emergency. Urgent orthopedic evaluation and treatment is essential to limit long-term disability.
2. Hemarthrosis indicates significant trauma (e.g., fracture or ligament disruption).

What are the admission criteria?

High clinical suspicion or other evidence of acute septic arthritis (i.e., fever, chills, or positive findings on joint fluid analysis)

OSTEOARTHRITIS (OA)

What is it?

Erosion of the cartilaginous articular surfaces of bones in any joint.

Osteophytes (jagged bony protrusions) usually form along the edges of the articular surfaces.

What is another term for OA?

Degenerative joint disease (DJD)

What causes it?

Trauma—due to repetitive microtrauma over many years or due to major traumatic joint injury

What are the common signs and symptoms?

Joint pain and swelling are the most common symptoms. Involved joints are usually not bilateral (i.e., they are asymmetric). Symptoms usually progress over months to years, although sudden increase in activity in an involved joint can lead to acute symptoms. Signs in the involved joint can vary greatly depending on severity of the disease; the joint may appear normal or it may show joint effusion, palpable osteophytes, and deformity.

What is unique about OA of the joints of the hand?

OA of the hands has a predilection to involve the distal interphalangeal (DIP) joints and a tendency to spare the proximal interphalangeal (PIP) and metacarpal-phalangeal (MCP) joints.

What are Heberden's nodes?

Hard, discrete nodules that form over the DIP joints in patients with OA

What tests are used to diagnose OA?

If a patient has a history and physical examination consistent with OA, other tests are not necessarily needed before beginning a therapeutic trial of medication (see below). Radiographs of the joint and synovial fluid analysis can help confirm the diagnosis in cases that are unclear.

What does the radiograph show in OA?

Osteophyte formation and narrowing of the joint space due to the erosion of articular cartilage.

What does joint fluid analysis show in OA?

Cell count of 200–300 WBC/μl
No crystals

Negative culture
Normal to mildly decreased viscosity

What physical or mechanical modalities are used to treat OA?

Heat before activity with ice after activity can decrease pain and swelling. Exercises that increase the strength of the muscles around the joint should be prescribed.

Decreasing the repetitive trauma across the involved joint (or joints) can be achieved by alterations in work activities or change to low-impact exercise programs (e.g., cycling, swimming).

What medications are used to treat OA?

NSAIDs have been the most common first-line agents, although studies have shown that acetaminophen can reduce pain to a similar degree. Injection of corticosteroids into the involved joint is also used occasionally.

Why have NSAIDs traditionally been used before acetaminophen in the treatment of OA?

It was thought that their anti-inflammatory effect would modify the disease process. However, studies have shown that NSAIDs do not alter the progression of OA. Therefore, acetaminophen is an acceptable alternative.

What are the most common side effects of NSAID use?

GI upset is the most common side effect. Gastric ulcers can complicate use of these agents and cause acute upper GI bleeding; this is more common in elderly patients. Increase in blood pressure is often seen with NSAID use and should be considered in patients with hypertension. Liver function abnormalities and renal impairment are less common, but significant, side effects in older patients.

What problems are associated with intra-articular corticosteroid injections?

Corticosteroids impair articular cartilage growth and repair. Therefore, overuse can accelerate progression of the disease process.

What surgical options are available for OA?

Osteophytes can be trimmed and intra-articular debris (calcified pieces of cartilage sheared from the articular surface) can be removed by arthroscopy. Experimental treatment using transplanted cartilage to fill in the erosions has shown promise. Joint replacement is reserved for patients with intractable pain or severe deformity.

RHEUMATOID ARTHRITIS (RA)

What is it?

An inflammatory arthritis characterized by synovial proliferation and progressive destruction of articular surfaces supporting ligaments and bone

What causes it?

It is thought to be secondary to an autoimmune process.

What are common signs and symptoms?

Joint pain, swelling, erythema, and effusion occur in a symmetrical pattern and are polyarticular (involve many joints). Symptoms tend to be worse in the morning and improve with use. Hands show involvement of the MCP joints with ulnar deviation of the fingers. Joint destruction and deformity can be profound and debilitating. Rheumatoid nodules can be present.

What are rheumatoid nodules?

Moderately sized (1–3 cm) nodules that are usually found on the extensor surface of the elbows

What tests are used to diagnose RA?

Serum test for rheumatoid factor (RF)
Erythrocyte sedimentation rate (ESR)
Joint fluid analysis
Radiography
CBC, ANA, and serum uric acid usually obtained to evaluate for other arthritides

What is the rheumatoid factor?

An antibody found in patients with RA thought to be one of the autoantibodies that cause the disease

What does joint fluid analysis reveal in patients with RA?

Cell count of 3,000–50,000 WBC/μl, decreased viscosity, no crystals, and a negative culture

What types of physical/ mechanical modalities are used to treat RA?	Heat can be very helpful, especially in the morning. Painful joints can be supported with splints or braces. Environmental alterations (e.g., extra-large handles for eating utensils) can also help the patient remain functional.
What are the three general types of therapy for RA?	Symptomatic therapy Remitting agents Palliation
What agents are used to control symptoms?	NSAIDs Corticosteroids
What agents are used to achieve remission of RA?	Methotrexate Gold 5-aminosalicylic acid (5-ASA)
How do these agents achieve remission?	They are immunosuppressant agents that are thought to suppress the production of autoantibodies.
What palliative measures are available?	Splints or braces may support severely affected joints to decrease pain. Joint replacement can be used in some cases. However, since RA is often polyarticular, replacing all involved joints can be impossible.
Helpful hints	1. Human lymphocyte antigen B27 (HLA-B27) is a genetic marker for patients with RA and other types of autoimmune diseases. 2. Remitting agents have the greatest benefit if started early in the course of the disease.

GOUTY ARTHRITIS (GOUT)

What is it?	A type of acute arthritis
What causes it?	Precipitation of uric acid crystals in the affected joint
What are common signs and symptoms of gout?	Severe pain with swelling and marked erythema of the involved joint. The joint is so tender that light touch (such as clothing or bed linens lying on it)

causes pain. The most commonly affected joint is the metatarsal-phalangeal joint of the great toe. Patients with advanced untreated cases can have gouty tophi.

What are gouty tophi?

Gouty tophi are subcutaneous nodules that are collections of uric acid crystals. They can occur anywhere and are sometimes difficult to distinguish from rheumatoid nodules.

What tests are used to evaluate gout?

Serum uric acid concentration
Joint fluid analysis
24-hour urinary excretion of uric acid

What does joint fluid analysis reveal in patients with gout?

Crystals that are negatively birefringent when examined under polarized light
Cell count of 3,000–50,000 WBC/μl
Negative culture

What agents are used to treat an acute episode of gout?

NSAIDs (usually indomethacin)
Colchicine
Corticosteroids (intra-articular or oral)

How is the chronic elevation of serum uric acid treated?

Decrease production of uric acid (allopurinol)
Increase urinary excretion of uric acid (probenecid and sulfinpyrazone)

How do the results of the 24-hour urinary excretion of uric acid help decide which agents to use to decrease uric acid concentrations?

If excretion is normal (800 mg of uric acid/24 hours or higher), the kidneys are attempting to excrete uric acid at a normal rate and cannot keep up with production. These patients are overproducers and are best treated with allopurinol.
If excretion is low (less than 800 mg of uric acid/24 hours), the kidney is not excreting uric acid quickly enough to keep serum concentrations normal. These patients are underexcreters and are best treated with uricosuric agents (probenecid or sulfinpyrazone).

What is the benefit of returning the uric acid level to normal?

Acute episodes of arthritis can be decreased in frequency and even eliminated in some cases. Long-term complications such as tophi and uric acid nephropathy can be avoided.

Helpful hints

1. Uric acid–lowering agents can make acute episodes worse. Therefore, do not initiate these agents until the acute episode is resolved.
2. Do not use ice on the involved joint even though there is marked erythema and warmth. Lower temperature will increase precipitation of crystals and make the episode worse.

FRACTURES

What are they?

A disruption or break in the cortex of a bone. By definition, in mature bone the disruption extends through the entire bone.

What is a closed fracture?

A fracture that occurs with the skin intact

What is an open fracture?

A fracture where the skin is opened, exposing the fracture to external microorganisms

What is the most common cause of fractures?

Trauma of a severe enough nature to cause disruption of an inherently strong support structure (i.e., bone)

What are other causes of fractures?

Repetitive minor trauma to a normally mineralized bone (stress fracture)

Minimal or insignificant trauma to a bone with underlying pathology such as inadequate mineralization (osteoporosis) or tumor infiltration (pathologic fracture)

What are common signs and symptoms of fracture?

Sudden onset of pain and swelling immediately after the traumatic event; pain is exacerbated by movement of, or bearing weight on, the affected bone

Deformity of the affected extremity

Open fractures will often have bone edges protruding from the wound.

What tests are used to diagnose fractures?	Plain radiographs of the injured area in multiple views (anterior/posterior, lateral, and oblique). Radionuclide bone scan or CT scan can be helpful in diagnosing stress fractures or traumatic fractures not identified with plain radiographs.
What is the first step in treatment of fractures?	Restoring the bone to normal (or near-normal) alignment (i.e., reducing the fracture), if needed.
What are the two ways this can be accomplished?	Closed reduction Open reduction
What is a closed reduction?	Manipulating the involved bone to restore normal alignment without resorting to surgery (i.e., the skin *is not* "opened").
What is an open reduction?	Using a surgical approach to affect proper alignment of the involved bone (i.e., the skin *is* "opened").
What is the second step in treating a fracture?	Immobilizing the fractured bone so that the proper alignment is maintained
What are the two ways this is accomplished?	1. External immobilization (cast or splint) 2. Internal fixation (using surgically placed rods, pins or screws to maintain proper alignment) followed by casting or splinting
How does one decide which approach to use to reduce or immobilize a fracture?	The nature of the trauma (e.g., penetrating versus nonpenetrating); the number of fragments of bone in the fracture area; and the blood supply, structure, and function of the involved bone are several of the important factors to consider in the decision of which approach to use. Open reduction is required for all open fractures so that the bone fragments can be debrided to decrease the risk of infection.
Helpful hints	1. Adequate anesthesia (local or regional) is essential before attempting closed reduction.

2. The vascular and neurological integrity of the involved extremity must be closely evaluated before and after reduction and immobilization.
3. The cast or splint should immobilize the joint above and below the fracture.

What are the admission criteria?

1. Parenteral analgesia required to control pain
2. Patients at high risk for vascular or neurological compromise such as severe soft tissue trauma, or patients who are post–open reduction or internal fixation
3. Patients at high risk for infection (open fractures)
4. Patients with multiple traumatic injuries requiring close monitoring and follow-up for other complications

TENDINITIS

What is it?

Inflammation of a tendon or tendon sheath

What causes it?

Tendinitis is caused by injury to the tendon, usually from overuse. The trauma is secondary to an increase in the forces borne across the tendon or repetitive motion across a bony prominence.

What are signs and symptoms of tendinitis?

Pain is the most common symptom, usually associated with a particular movement that stresses the involved tendon. Palpation over the involved tendon will reproduce pain. Occasionally, swelling in the tendon can be palpated, but there is no joint swelling or effusion.

What diagnostic tests are used with tendinitis?

Usually none. The history and physical examination are enough to diagnose the majority of cases.

How is tendinitis treated?

Heat before activity and ice after activity (helpful to control pain)

NSAIDs
Alteration of activities (work or
 recreational) that cause symptoms

LIGAMENTOUS SPRAINS (SPRAINS)

What are they?
 Stretch injuries to the ligaments of any
joint

What causes them?
 Acute trauma that causes the ligament to
stretch beyond its limit of elasticity

**What are common signs
and symptoms of sprains?**
 Acute pain and swelling of the involved
joint are present to varying degrees.
Joint effusion is often present, and there
is focal tenderness over the involved
ligament. The joint usually has some
degree of instability when stress forces
are applied during examination.

**How are sprains graded
and what do the grades
mean?**

1. First-degree sprain: The ligament has
   a minimal stretch injury. Pain and
   swelling may be present but the joint
   has little or no laxity.
2. Second-degree sprain: The ligament
   is moderately injured. Pain and
   swelling are present and the joint has
   some laxity when stressed, but a
   definite end point of laxity is felt on
   examination.
3. Third-degree sprain: The ligament is
   completely disrupted (torn). Marked
   pain and swelling are usually present
   and the joint is unstable.

**What diagnostic tests are
used?**
 Radiographs (often obtained to rule out
fracture)
Joint fluid analysis
MRI or arthrogram (can assist in
diagnosing cases where surgical repair
is being considered)

**What does joint fluid
analysis show with severe
sprains?**
 Hemarthrosis

How are sprains treated?
 General measure—*r*est, *i*ce,
*c*ompression, *e*levation (RICE).
NSAIDs are often used as analgesics.

Splinting—provides support for unstable joints and prevents recurrence of stretch

Surgical repair—third-degree sprains of joints where full function is needed (e.g., knee, ankle)

Helpful hints

1. Lower extremity sprains may require the patient to use crutches if unable to bear weight comfortably.
2. It is important to investigate functional requirements for the patient's job. This information may lead to a more aggressive therapeutic approach (e.g., a third-degree sprain of a lateral collateral ligament of the PIP joint may need surgical repair if the patient requires full function of the involved finger in his or her work).

What are the admission criteria?

1. In the case of a major injury to a large joint where IV pain medication may be required
2. If the injury is severe enough that it may lead to large hemarthroses (blood in the joint), which can occasionally cause hypotension

12   Common Neurologic Problems

CEREBROVASCULAR DISEASE (CVD)

What is it?	A variety of disorders of the arteries that supply blood to the brain
What are the most common causes of CVD?	Atherosclerosis Hypertension Aneurysm Vasculitis Infection
What are the risk factors for CVD?	Hypertension Smoking Hypercholesterolemia Diabetes mellitus Family history Atherosclerotic vascular disease in other organs (e.g., coronary artery disease)
What are the common clinical syndromes of CVD?	Cerebrovascular accident (CVA) Transient ischemic attack (TIA)
What is a CVA?	A vascular event in the brain that causes a neurologic deficit
What are the three causes of CVAs?	Ischemia Intracerebral hemorrhage (ICH) Subarachnoid hemorrhage (SAH)
What is a TIA?	A neurologic deficit caused by an ischemic event where the neurologic deficit resolves spontaneously in less than 24 hours
What are clinical characteristics of ischemic events (CVAs, TIAs)?	Neurologic deficits may wax and wane or gradually progress. There may be worsening or complete resolution of

symptoms with time. There is often a preceding "warning" event.

What causes ischemic cerebrovascular events?

Spontaneous thrombosis ($\frac{2}{3}$)
Thromboembolism ($\frac{1}{3}$)

What are the most common sources of thromboembolism?

Thromboses in the heart that occur secondary to arrhythmias
Thromboses from ulcerated plaques in the carotid arteries

What is the most common arrhythmia associated with thromboembolism?

Atrial fibrillation

What are the clinical characteristics of an intracerebral hemorrhage?

Sudden onset of neurologic deficits that do not fluctuate with time
Usually no preceding "warning" event

What is the most common cause of ICH?

Hypertension

How does it occur?

The penetrating vessels of the basal ganglia are weakened by chronic hypertension, allowing small aneurysms to form. The weakened vessel or the aneurysm can rupture, resulting in bleeding into the brain tissue.

What are the clinical characteristics of subarachnoid hemorrhage?

Sudden onset of severe headache (classically described by the patient as, "The worst headache of my life")
Nuchal rigidity
Altered mental status

What are the most common causes of SAH?

Berry aneurysms of surface arteries
Arteriovenous (AV) malformations

What are common signs and symptoms of CVD?

Altered mental status
Weakness
Numbness
Speech difficulties
Visual difficulties
Dizziness
Bruits over extracranial arteries
Headache
Muscle weakness (plegia) or paralysis (paresis)

Sensory deficits

Loss of deep tendon reflexes

Coordination difficulties

Abnormal gait

Romberg sign

Babinski sign

Muscle tone absent or diminished in acute phase of event, but hyperactive later

How are these symptoms distinguished from other neurologic problems?

In CVA, signs and symptoms occur in patterns that are referable to the area of the brain affected by the event.

What laboratory tests are used to evaluate patients with an acute CVA?

CBC

Prothrombin and partial thromboplastin times

Erythrocyte sedimentation rate

Spinal fluid analysis

ECG

Echocardiogram

EEG

Serum electrolytes

What radiologic study is used to evaluate patients with an acute CVA?

CT scan without contrast

Why?

It reliably identifies hemorrhage (both ICH and SAH), it is easier to perform (takes less time and less patient cooperation) than MRI, and it is cheaper than MRI. Ischemic CVAs often are not identified by CT or MRI early in the course of the event; ischemia takes time to alter the structure of the brain to where it can be identified with imaging.

Why is it important to identify hemorrhagic versus ischemic CVA?

The treatment is different for hemorrhage than for ischemia CVA.

How are ischemic CVAs treated?

If the patient presents within 3 hours after onset of symptoms, thrombolytics are considered. Otherwise, supportive care is provided: aspirin is given, blood pressure is maintained in the high-normal range (i.e., blood pressue is not excessively lowered with medication), nutritional support is given if necessary, and early rehabilitation is initiated. A patient with posterior circulation ischemia, documented cardiac thrombus, or a fluctuating neurologic deficit should be considered for anticoagulation with heparin followed by warfarin.

How are hemorrhagic CVAs treated?

Clotting abnormalities are corrected, blood pressure is maintained in the low-normal range, and nutritional support (if necessary) and early rehabilitation are provided. Intracranial pressure is monitored as indicated by the clinical course. With SAH, surgery is indicated to tie off aneurysms or AV malformations before they can bleed again. With ICH, surgical drainage can be considered depending on the clinical situation (size of bleed, accessibility of lesion, long-term neurologic consequences).

How can CVAs be prevented?

Risk factor modification
Control of hypertension
Aspirin
Prophylactic warfarin in patients with atrial fibrillation
Treatment of early ischemic CVD (i.e., before a CVA occurs)

How is treatable early CVD identified?

Identifying and evaluating TIAs
Monitoring for carotid bruits

What diagnostic tests are used to evaluate carotid bruit with or without TIA, and what is the role of each test?

Carotid duplex ultrasound with Doppler—evaluates for significant stenosis (> 70%) and/or ulceration of the plaque in the extracranial arteries (common carotid and proximal internal carotid) that would indicate a high risk of a CVA
Carotid angiogram—identifies anatomy for surgical intervention
MRI or CT—identifies presence or extent of previous small, subclinical ischemic infarcts (lacunar infarcts)

How is early CVD in the extracranial vessels treated?	Surgical endarterectomy should be considered for significant lesions of the carotid artery, especially in patients with symptoms or evidence of ischemic events (TIA, lacunar infarcts). Risk factors are aggressively modified (e.g., hypertension is controlled, cholesterol is lowered).
What are the admission criteria?	1. Unstable or fluctuating neurologic deficit 2. New onset CVA until the patient is stable 3. Hemodynamic instability

CARPAL TUNNEL SYNDROME

What is it?	A clinical syndrome secondary to dysfunction of the distal median nerve
What causes it?	Increased pressure in the carpal tunnel of the wrist disrupts the normal function of the median nerve as it enters the hand.
What are the risk factors?	Occupations or hobbies that require repetitive motion of the hand or wrist Previous trauma to the wrist, especially fractures Diabetes mellitus Autoimmune diseases Obesity
What are the common symptoms?	Numbness and tingling in the thumb, index, and middle fingers Weakness of the hand Pain of the wrist and hand Referred pain to the elbow and/or shoulder The pain and numbness are usually worse at night, causing awakening and usually inducing the patient to shake the hand(s) to relieve symptoms.
What are the common physical findings?	Weakness of the intrinsic muscles of the hand

	Impaired sensation of the thumb, index, and middle fingers Reproduction of symptoms with extreme flexion of the wrist Reproduction of symptoms with tapping over the ventral aspect of the wrist (Tinel's sign) Wasting of the thenar eminence (with long-standing disease)
What diagnostic test confirms median nerve dysfunction in the carpal tunnel?	Nerve conduction studies of the involved extremity
How is carpal tunnel syndrome treated?	NSAIDs Wrist splints, especially at night Workstation evaluation to modify repetitive movements that aggravate symptoms Corticosteroid injection into the carpal tunnel Surgical release of the flexor retinaculum that forms the roof of the carpal tunnel
Which patients require nerve conduction studies?	Those unresponsive to conservative therapy who are contemplating surgery
Helpful hint	Nocturnal hand-shaking is the most reliable clinical indicator of carpal tunnel syndrome.

DEMENTIA

What is it?	Progressive loss of cognitive function that interferes with work or social functioning. It usually has an insidious onset. Initial manifestation is memory impairment. The level of consciousness is not impaired.
What are the causes of dementia?	Idiopathic (no identifiable cause) Cerebrovascular disease Space-occupying brain lesion (e.g., tumor) Infection (neurosyphilis, cryptococcus) Normal pressure hydrocephalus

Hypothyroidism
Vitamin B$_{12}$ deficiency
Depression
Drugs

What is the term for idiopathic dementia?

Alzheimer's disease

What are common signs and symptoms of dementia?

Impaired memory (especially short-term memory) and judgment
Wandering
Confusion
Decline in ability to perform basic mathematics
Incontinence
Neurologic examination findings can be normal or consistent with any of the diseases listed above.

What is the main goal of the diagnostic evaluation of dementia?

To identify patients who have a treatable cause of their dementia

What tests are used to evaluate patients with dementia?

Blood tests—CBC, ESR, TSH, glucose, electrolytes, syphilis serology, and vitamin B$_{12}$ level
Spinal fluid analysis—cerebrospinal fluid pressure, India ink stain, and syphilis serology in addition to the routine cell counts, culture, and protein and glucose levels
Brain imaging with CT or MRI—indicated in patients with focal neurologic deficits, but its utility is controversial in patients with normal neurologic examination findings owing to low yield in finding treatable problems

How is dementia treated?

Treat the underlying cause, if one is identified.
Provide supportive care for the patient and family (especially in the case of Alzheimer's disease) to assure patient safety and to help the family cope with the difficult challenges.
Tacrine or donapazil can help some patients with Alzheimer's dementia,

but therapeutic benefit is usually transient (there is an average of 6 months' delay in progression).

Helpful hints

1. Recently identified genetic indicators for Alzheimer's disease may provide insight into etiology and potential treatments.
2. Long-term nursing-home care is often required as dementia progresses. Incontinence, aggressive behavior, or wandering are often the precipitating factors for families to consider nursing home placement.
3. Because the family will have many issues to deal with, support groups may be helpful.

What are the admission criteria?

When family resources (time, emotional resources) become overwhelmed or when the patient is no longer safe in the home environment, admission to a nursing facility is indicated.

TENSION HEADACHE

What is it?

A pain in the head thought to be secondary to increased tone in the muscles of the head or neck

What causes it?

Psychosocial stress, depression, or anxiety

What other syndromes can produce headaches similar to tension headaches?

Chronic fatigue syndrome
Fibromyalgia
Localized myositis
Chronic sinusitis
Common migraine
Temporomandibular joint (TMJ) syndrome

What are common signs and symptoms of tension headaches?

The pain classically begins in the occipital region of the head and spreads around the sides of the head in a bandlike manner. The patient often describes a pressure sensation as though the head were in a vise. Neurologic examination findings are normal, but there is often increased tone and tenderness along the occiput, neck muscles, and temporalis muscle. Acute or chronic life stressors are frequently identified.

What diagnostic tests are indicated in a patient with tension headaches?

None. When a patient has a history and physical examination findings consistent with tension headache, no further tests are needed.

How are tension headaches treated?

Analgesia
Stress management
Counseling
Treatment of underlying anxiety disorder (if one exists; see Chapter 15)

Helpful hints

1. Acetaminophen and NSAIDs are analgesics of choice. Use narcotics with great caution.
2. Follow patient closely. If patient does not respond to treatment, re-evaluate to see if new signs or symptoms are present.
3. Stress is caused by change, even positive change. Patients complaining of tension headaches may be experiencing many new positive events in their lives and deny that they have stress, not realizing that positive changes can increase stress levels as much as negative events.

MIGRAINE HEADACHE

What is it?

Head pain that is thought to be secondary to neurovascular and neurohormonal changes in the brain

What are some of the common triggers?

Foods containing vasoactive substances (e.g., caffeine, red wine, aged cheese)
Menstrual or premenstrual hormonal changes
Fasting and stress (physical or psychological)

What are the common symptoms?

An aura followed by a unilateral throbbing headache
Photophobia
Nausea or vomiting

What is an aura?

A symptom complex that begins and resolves just prior to the onset of the symptoms diagnostic of an illness. The characteristics of an aura are usually of a neurologic nature (e.g., visual field change, focal numbness or weakness). In migraine headaches, the symptom complex occurs and resolves just before the onset of headache.

What is the most common aura for migraine headache?

Visual scotoma

What is a visual scotoma?

An alteration of the visual pathway experienced by patients as squiggly lines or a cloud that obscures all or a portion of the visual field

What are migraine headaches with an aura called?

Classic migraines

What are migraine headaches without an aura called?

Common migraines

What are the physical findings in a patient with migraine headache?

The patient appears to be in significant pain, will avoid light, and will sometimes vomit. Otherwise, the examination findings are usually normal.

What diagnostic tests are performed on patients with migraine headache?

Usually none. Some practitioners will argue that a patient with new-onset migraine headaches should undergo a CT scan to rule out other intracranial pathology. However, a CT scan is usually not indicated if the symptoms are consistent with migraine headache and if the neurologic examination findings are normal.

How are migraine headaches treated?

Sumatriptan
Analgesics
Antiemetics

What migraine headache symptoms often complicate therapy?	Nausea and vomiting often require that therapy be administered parenterally.
Can migraine headaches be prevented?	Yes. There are drugs that, if taken regularly (daily), can decrease the frequency of migraine headaches.
What drugs are commonly used for migraine headache prophylaxis?	Tricyclic antidepressants β-adrenergic blockers Calcium channel blockers
Helpful hints	1. Sumatriptan therapy can precipitate vascular events (MI, CVA). Therefore, it should be administered in the office the first time it is used in a patient. 2. IM sumatriptan is more effective than the oral form.

SEIZURES

What are they?	Unorganized electrical activity in the brain. This unorganized electrical activity can affect a focal area of the cortex (partial seizures) or the entire cortex (generalized seizures).
What is the old medical term (now often used by the general public) for a seizure disorder?	Epilepsy
What causes seizures?	Scar tissue in the brain (congenital, traumatic, CVA) Fever Infection Drugs, especially overdoses and drugs of abuse (alcohol, cocaine) Acute trauma (closed or penetrating) Metabolic abnormalities Cerebrovascular events Tumors
What are the signs and symptoms of generalized seizures?	Diffuse tonic/clonic activity (unorganized shaking or jerking) of the extremities and trunk is the most common finding. Sometimes, generalized seizures will

disrupt only cognitive abilities and will not have motor manifestations (absence seizures). Decreased alertness is often seen for 15 to 30 minutes after the seizure activity ceases. The patient may bite the tongue and may be incontinent of stool or urine. The patient will not be able to remember the event but may recall an aura just prior to losing consciousness. Transient neurologic abnormalities (e.g., downgoing toes on Babinski test, focal weakness) can be found on examination in the immediate postictal period.

What is the term used to describe the altered mental alertness after a generalized seizure?

Postictal state

What are the symptoms of focal seizures?

Tonic/clonic activity in one extremity, visual hallucinations, lip smacking, unusual aromas, or sudden changes in behavior. Auras are common. Neurologic findings are less common, and mental status changes after the seizure are often absent.

How long do seizures last?

Most last for a few seconds to a few minutes and respond promptly to treatment.

What is prolonged seizure activity unresponsive to initial therapy called?

Status epilepticus

What diagnostic tests are used with seizures?

Electroencephalogram (EEG)—This is the gold standard for diagnosis. The EEG can be monitored over long periods of time, if necessary, to document seizure activity.
Laboratory tests—CBC, serum electrolytes, serum calcium, serum magnesium, serum alcohol level, urine drug screen, serum levels of suspected overdose drugs, serum levels of antiepileptic drugs, arterial blood gas, and lumbar puncture with cerebrospinal fluid analysis
Imaging—CT scan or MRI

Laboratory tests and radiographic images are evaluated to attempt to identify an etiology for the seizure.

How are active seizures or status epilepticus treated?

Diazepam, lorazepam, phenytoin or phenobarbital, administered IV, are used as first-line agents. Correction of metabolic abnormalities (hypoxia, hypotension, lactic acidosis, myoglobinuria, etc.) and initiating treatment of other problems that cause seizures (see above) are indicated. Occasionally, status epilepticus requires general anesthesia to stop tonic/clonic movements.

What agents are commonly used to prevent recurrence of seizures?

Phenytoin
Phenobarbital
Carbamazepine
Valproic acid

Why is therapy with these agents often complicated?

The serum level of the drug must be maintained in a narrow therapeutic range. A little too much drug can cause serious side effects, while not enough drug can lead to recurrent seizures. Serum drug levels must be followed carefully.

What is the goal of therapy?

To prevent all seizures

Is this a realistic goal?

In most cases, yes. However, some seizure disorders are recalcitrant to treatment; in such cases, attempting to minimize the frequency of seizures is the goal of treatment.

What is the public health issue for persons with seizure disorders?

Operation of motor vehicles or other machinery that could harm the patient or others if the person with the seizure disorder has a seizure and loses control of the vehicle or machine.

Are health professionals required to report persons with seizure disorders to public health authorities?

This requirement varies from state to state. However, health professionals do have a duty to prevent persons without good seizure control from operating machinery that could be dangerous to themselves or others.

Helpful hints

1. Persons with well-controlled seizure disorders can live a normal life with no restrictions on activities.
2. Certain drugs are more effective for certain types of seizures (as identified clinically or on EEG).
3. Simple febrile seizures in children seldom indicate a long-term problem and do not require extensive evaluation (lumbar puncture, cultures, CT, etc.) if a source of the fever is readily identified (e.g., otitis media, upper respiratory illness).
4. Know the reporting requirements for your state.

What are the admission criteria?

1. Status epilepticus
2. Overdose or drug withdrawal situations
3. Acute trauma or CVA with seizure
4. Metabolic abnormalities that don't quickly correct with treatment
5. Central nervous system infections
6. New-onset seizures of unclear etiology

VERTIGO

What is it?

The subjective feeling that the environment is spinning around. It is often described as dizziness or feeling "off balance."

What are the causes? (Give examples of each.)

Inner ear disease (examples—labyrinthitis, Meniere's disease, benign positional vertigo)
Tumor (example—acoustic neuroma)
Posterior circulation cerebrovascular disease (example—vertebrobasilar insufficiency)
Drugs (example—phenytoin)

What other symptoms frequently accompany vertigo?

Nausea
Vomiting
Tinnitus

Hearing loss
Difficulty walking
Intolerance of motion (e.g., riding in a
car)

What is the classic triad of symptoms in Meniere's disease?

Vertigo
Tinnitus
Bilateral hearing loss

What physical findings are important in patients with vertigo?

Nystagmus
Middle ear effusion
Positive Romberg test
Abnormalities of strength, sensation,
gait, or coordination
Reproduction of symptoms with
provocative testing (rapid changes in
head position by the examiner)
Hearing loss (especially if unilateral)

What tests are used in patients with vertigo?

Audiometry, CT scan, MRI, and
angiography are considered, depending
on the clinical picture.

How is vertigo treated?

As with most problems, it is best treated
by treating the underlying cause, if
possible. Acute severe vertigo will often
respond to diazepam. Inner ear
problems are the most common cause of
vertigo, and the symptoms will usually
respond to meclizine, cyclizine, or
dimenhydrinate. A low salt diet or
diuretics may help patients with
Meniere's disease. Vertebrobasilar
insufficiency is treated with aspirin or
warfarin. Drugs can be adjusted or
discontinued. Tumors are treated by
surgical resection or radiation.

13

Common Prenatal Issues in the Primary Care Setting

This chapter covers prenatal issues that present to primary care offices for evaluation and management, even if the primary care provider does not regularly administer prenatal care. This chapter is not meant to cover all prenatal issues that arise in a family practice or obstetrics and gynecology office that provides ongoing prenatal care.

DIAGNOSIS OF PREGNANCY

Why is this important?

The whole approach to a patient changes if she is pregnant. The medications used, tests ordered, and medical and psychological implications of symptoms are much different in the pregnant versus the nonpregnant patient. Determine the estimated gestational age (EGA) early, because this increases accuracy. If the pregnancy is unplanned, address all issues early, especially if the patient desires termination.

What are the symptoms of pregnancy?

Amenorrhea is the most common symptom, but it is not always present or recognized (e.g., implantation bleeding may occur at the time of the next expected menstrual period). Breast enlargement and tenderness, morning nausea, fatigue, vaginal bleeding, and pelvic pain are other common symptoms associated with pregnancy.

What is the key to diagnosing pregnancy?

Presence of beta human chorionic gonadotropin (β-HCG) in the urine or serum of the patient

How long after conception can β-HCG be detected?	In serum, 4–5 days In urine, 6–8 days (first-void morning specimen is best)
Why is the first-void morning urine specimen preferred when diagnosing pregnancy?	Because most people do not void during the night, substances filtrated by the kidneys accumulate in the bladder. Because β-HCG is filtered by the kidneys, it is expected to accumulate in the bladder throughout the night and thus have a higher concentration in a first-voided morning specimen. This possibility increases the likelihood of detecting low levels of β-HCG early in pregnancy.
What are the two serum tests for β-HCG?	1. Qualitative β-HCG: confirms presence of β-HCG in serum 2. Quantitative β-HCG: determines the concentration of β-HCG in serum
In what situations is qualitative β-HCG used?	It is used to diagnose pregnancy when the clinical suspicion is high, but the urine test is negative. It is usually used very early in the pregnancy. [**Note:** Some physicians continue to think that the serum β-HCG can be detected much earlier than urine β-HCG, because first-generation urine tests were only positive after 6 weeks of pregnancy. However, the modern office and over-the-counter (OTC) tests used to detect β-HCG in urine will detect β-HCG only 2–4 days after it is detectable in the serum.]
In what situations is quantitative β-HCG used?	It is used when the β-HCG concentration is needed for clinical decision making (e.g., threatened abortion, suspected fetal demise without bleeding).
How quickly does the β-HCG concentration increase in a normal pregnancy?	It doubles every 48–72 hours.
What role does ultrasound have in diagnosing pregnancy?	In most cases, none. It can help establish the location (e.g., intrauterine versus ectopic) and viability of the

pregnancy, but the ultrasound cannot detect pregnancy until about 5 weeks EGA, which is long after the urine and serum β-HCG tests are positive.

DRUG THERAPY IN THE PREGNANT PATIENT

What is the issue?

Prescription and OTC drugs are commonly used. And, because of the growth and tissue differentiation of the developing embryo/fetus, it is extremely susceptible to drug effects that may not be apparent in the adult population that uses them.

What essential property must a drug have to affect the developing embryo/fetus?

It must cross the placenta, so that it moves from the maternal to the fetal circulation.

When is the fetus most susceptible to drugs that affect organ or tissue differentiation?

During the first trimester—most organs and tissues have undergone differentiation by the 12th week, so most gross physical abnormalities (e.g., limb abnormalities cause by thalidomide) occur early in pregnancy regardless of whether the cause is genetic or drug-related.

Do drugs have other adverse effects later in the pregnancy?

Yes. Drugs may have many metabolic effects that can affect normal growth and development of the fetus.

How can one find out which drugs are prohibited in pregnant patients?

All drugs have a pregnancy category rating in their product information.

What is the pregnancy rating?

Drugs are classified as A, B, C, D, or X, depending on the information available to determine their safety.

What does each class indicate?
    Class A?

The drug has been shown in clinical trials to be safe for use in pregnancy.

    Class B?

The drug has been shown to be safe in pregnancy in animal models; or, if adverse effects occurred in animal studies, they were not confirmed in human studies.

Class C?

The drug has shown adverse effects in animal studies, or there are no human or animal studies available. Risks and benefits should be weighed before a pregnant woman uses it.

Class D?

The drugs has shown adverse effects in human studies, but the benefits to the pregnant woman might outweigh the risks in a serious medical situation.

Class X?

The drug has been shown to cause adverse effects in pregnancy and this risk clearly outweighs any benefit. The drug should never be used in pregnant patients.

Helpful hints

1. A great resource is *Drugs in Pregnancy and Lactation* by Briggs, Freeman, and Yaffe (Williams & Wilkins, 1994).
2. Always check the pregnancy category before prescribing drugs to pregnant patients.
3. Determine the pregnancy status of all women in child-bearing years before prescribing medication.
4. Because most drugs have not been studied in clinical trials to determine safety in pregnancy, most categories are a "best guess" estimate of risk.

(**Note:** Most of these issues also apply to women who breast-feed their babies.)

DATING OF PREGNANCY

What is it?

Determining the EGA of the fetus and the estimated date of delivery (EDD)

Why is it important?

Because many prenatal care interventions and screens depend on accurate dating; also, if problems arise that necessitate delivery, knowledge of gestational age helps maximize the chances for favorable outcomes for both mother and baby.

How long is a normal pregnancy?

40 weeks, or 280 days, from the last normal menstrual period (LNMP)

What are three commonly used methods of dating?

1. Time from a reliable LNMP is considered the most accurate method of dating:
   Pregnancy calculators (wheels) can be used.
   Nägele's rule: Subtract 3 months from the LNMP month and add 7 days to the first day of the LNMP (assumes a 28-day cycle).
2. Clinical parameters:
   Uterine size: 8 weeks = palpable at symphysis pubis; 15 weeks = halfway between pubis and umbilicus; 20 weeks = umbilicus
   Fetal heart beat: audible with Doppler at around 10 weeks
   Quickening (i.e., mother's first sensation of fetal movement): 18–20 weeks in a primipara; 17 weeks in a multipara
3. Fetal ultrasound:
   Measurement of the biparietal diameter is very accurate at around 20 weeks.
   Greater than 30 weeks dating by ultrasound can have a $+/-$ 2 weeks error.
   Ultrasound is relied on when the LNMP is uncertain.

NAUSEA IN PREGNANCY

What is morning sickness?

Nausea (and sometimes vomiting) that occurs in the first trimester of pregnancy

How common is nausea in pregnancy?

Approximately 50% of all pregnancies are complicated by nausea.

What causes it?

The exact etiology is unclear, but it seems partially associated with the rapid increase in β-HCG serum levels early in pregnancy.

At what point during pregnancy are the symptoms most prominent?	Between 2 and 12 weeks EGA; symptoms usually occur in the morning
What are two precipitating factors?	Emotional stress and strong odors
What tests are performed on patients with nausea of pregnancy?	Urinalysis (specific gravity and ketones most applicable) and serum electrolytes are used to check for fluid status, ketosis, and/or electrolyte abnormalities. In severe cases, ultrasound is considered to evaluate for molar pregnancy and/or multiple gestation.
How is it treated?	Eating light, dry foods (e.g., crackers) Eating frequent, small meals Emotional support Vitamin B_6 is sometimes helpful. Antinausea drugs are used as a last resort measure.
What is hyperemesis gravidarum?	Extreme nausea and vomiting during pregnancy associated with ketonuria and dehydration
How is it treated?	It often requires IV fluids, parenteral medications for emesis control, and electrolyte monitoring.
What are the admission criteria for a pregnant patient with nausea?	Unrelenting nausea and vomiting with dehydration, electrolyte abnormalities, or nutritional compromise (marked weight loss)
Helpful hints	1. Closely observe patients with nausea for weight loss and/or nutritional compromise that could impair fetal growth. 2. Hyperemesis may be a sign of molar pregnancy or multiple gestation.

BLEEDING IN PREGNANCY

What is it?	Vaginal bleeding before delivery of the infant; it is distinct from postpartum hemorrhage

During which trimesters is bleeding most common?

The first and third trimesters

In what percent of pregnancies does the woman have bleeding in the first trimester?

25%

What are the causes of first trimester bleeding?

Spontaneous abortion
Implantation of fetus
Trauma
Ectopic pregnancy
Unknown etiology

What are the causes of third trimester bleeding?

Placenta previa
Placental abruption
Uterine rupture
Fetal vessel rupture
Cervical or vaginal laceration/lesion
Coagulopathies

What are important historical factors in evaluating patients with bleeding in pregnancy?

Time of onset
Amount of bleeding
Recent abdominal trauma
Contractions
Date of last intercourse
Gestational age (which should be established as accurately as possible)
History of cesarean section, placenta previa, or coagulation disorder

What are important physical findings?

1. **Vital signs,** including fetal heart rate and the amount of bleeding, must be established first. This information delineates how aggressively supportive therapy needs to be instituted and at what pace diagnostic procedures and/ or consultation should proceed. Look for other sites of bleeding and associated signs, such as petechiae.
2. The **abdominal exam** should focus on uterine size and any tenderness.
3. Generally, the **pelvic examination** is deferred until placenta previa is ruled out by ultrasound (especially if the patient is near term). If placenta previa is ruled out, a sterile speculum exam may be performed to look for any mass or laceration and to check cervical dilatation.

What laboratory studies should be ordered?	CBC with platelets Blood type and Rh Serum β-HCG (quantitative only) Serum liver enzymes Kleihauer-Betke test (detects fetal RBCs in the maternal circulation) Prothrombin time (PT) Partial thromboplastin time (PTT)
What is the most common imaging technique used?	Ultrasound
What are the general principles of treatment for bleeding in pregnancy?	As with bleeding of any cause, a rapid but thorough history and physical exam must accompany adequate IV access and appropriate laboratory testing (including a hematocrit, platelet count, coagulation studies, and a type and screen should transfusion be necessary). Definitive treatment depends on the etiology of the bleeding.
What are the admission criteria for bleeding in pregnancy? **First trimester bleeding?**	Admit any patient with evidence of excessive bleeding, hemodynamic compromise, incomplete abortion, or ectopic pregnancy.
Third trimester bleeding?	All patients with third trimester bleeding should be admitted for observation and evaluation, because all causes of third-trimester bleeding are potentially life threatening to the patient and/or fetus.

SPONTANEOUS ABORTION

What is it?	An unplanned loss of the fetus in the first trimester (equivalent to the lay term *miscarriage*)
What are the five classifications of spontaneous abortion?	1. Threatened abortion 2. Inevitable abortion 3. Incomplete abortion 4. Complete abortion 5. Missed abortion

Define threatened abortion.

Vaginal bleeding without pain at less than 20 weeks' gestation with a closed cervical os

How is it evaluated?

Evaluate with serum β-HCG and ultrasound. If cardiac activity is detected, there is a > 90% chance the patient will go to term.

How is it managed?

Because no intervention has shown to affect outcomes, manage as outpatient with close follow-up.

Define an inevitable abortion.

Vaginal bleeding, cramping pelvic pain, and partially open cervical os with evidence of a viable fetus by ultrasound

How is it evaluated?

Evaluate with CBC, serum β-HCG, and ultrasound.

How is it managed?

Manage the patient in the hospital with pain control, and see if it becomes a complete or incomplete abortion.

Define an incomplete abortion.

Vaginal bleeding, cramping pelvic pain, and partially open cervical os without evidence of a viable fetus and with retained products of conception by ultrasound

How is it evaluated?

Evaluate with ultrasound and serum β-HCG. Consider CBC, blood type with antibody screen, PT, and PTT.

How is it managed?

Manage the patient in the hospital with supportive care, and evacuate products of conception surgically with dilatation and curettage (D&C). These patients must be followed closely, because most of them are prone to complications [e.g., septic abortion, disseminated intravascular coagulation (DIC)].

Define a complete abortion.

Vaginal bleeding and pain stop, all products of conception are passed, the cervical os closes, and the serum β-HCG becomes negative. No further medical treatment is needed.

Define a missed abortion.	The fetus dies but is retained without bleeding or passage of products of conception (can be for prolonged periods).
How is it evaluated?	Evaluation is by ultrasound identification of fetal demise and serum β-HCG decreasing to zero.
How is it managed?	Occasionally, these cases are managed with close follow-up to give the patient time to complete abortion spontaneously. However, if evidence of complications occurs, if spontaneous process does not begin in 10 to 14 days, or if patient wants to complete the process immediately, surgical evacuation by D&C is indicated.

Helpful hints

1. Be certain to administer Rh immune globulin if the patient is Rh negative.
2. Many factors are involved in spontaneous abortion, but the most common are nonrepeating chromosomal abnormalities leading to a nonviable fetus.
3. Offer support and allow the patient and/or partner to express emotions associated with the loss. You cannot overemphasize that nothing they did or did not do caused this; nothing they did or did not do could prevent this.
4. Recurrent abortions (> 3) are a special topic. The patient requires further evaluation to exclude infections, systemic disease, and/or chromosomal abnormalities.
5. Address the issue of future fertility.

ECTOPIC PREGNANCY

What is it?	Implantation and growth of an embryo outside the uterus
What is the most common location for an ectopic pregnancy?	The fallopian tube

What are the risk factors for ectopic pregnancy?

History of:
Pelvic inflammatory disease (increases risk from 0.5% to 4%)
Previous ectopic pregnancy
Tubal ligation or reconstruction in last 1 to 2 years
IUD (previously or currently in place)

What is the classic triad of symptoms?

Abdominal pain (90%)
Vaginal bleeding (50%–80%)
Amenorrhea (75%–90%)

What physical findings indicate ectopic pregnancy?

Low abdominal tenderness with adnexal tenderness are the most common findings; sometimes an adnexal mass may be palpated.

What two diagnostic tests are used to detect ectopic pregnancy?

Ultrasound and serum β-HCG

How is the ultrasound used to diagnose ectopic pregnancy?

Transvaginal ultrasound can detect intrauterine pregnancy (IUP) by 5 weeks; if IUP is identified, ectopic pregnancy can likely be excluded (coexisting IUP and ectopic occur 1 in 30,000 gestations).

How is ectopic pregnancy treated?

Surgical removal of the ectopic pregnancy is the most common method used. The procedure can be done laparoscopically for small ectopics (< 3 cm). Some advocate medical ablation of the pregnancy with methotrexate.

What are potential complications of untreated ectopic pregnancy?

Rupture of fallopian tube, with potential for massive internal hemorrhage and death

What are the admission criteria for a patient with an ectopic pregnancy?

All patients with a high suspicion for or documented ectopic pregnancy should be admitted and monitored closely in concert with an OB/GYN consult until surgery is performed.

Helpful hints

1. The incidence of ectopic pregnancy has been increasing over the last 20 years.

2. It is the leading cause of maternal mortality in the first trimester.

PLACENTA PREVIA

What is it?	The placenta is located on or adjacent to the cervical os.
What is the incidence of placenta previa?	0.5%
What percent of antepartum hemorrhages are caused by placenta previa?	20%
What are risk factors for placenta previa?	Multiparity Increasing maternal age Multiple gestations Previous previa
What are the three grades of placenta previa?	Complete—placenta covers the os Partial—placenta partially covers the os Marginal—placenta is next to the os
What are the signs and symptoms?	The classic presentation is *painless* vaginal bleeding (70%). Uterine contractions are present in 20% of cases.
What diagnostic tests are used?	Ultrasound is used to identify the location of the placenta. CBC with platelets, liver enzymes, PT, and PTT are used to evaluate severity of blood loss and potential complications.
How is placenta previa treated?	Stabilize patient and fetus with general measures for bleeding in pregnancy. If the pregnancy is at term, the bleeding is profuse, and/or patient remains unstable, then deliver by cesarean section immediately. If the patient and fetus are stable and preterm, attempt bed rest and follow hematocrit until term. Then, deliver by cesarean section because elective deliveries pose less risk for mother and child (tocolysis is safe if concomitant abruption has been excluded).

Helpful hints

1. Rh-negative patients need the Kleihauer-Betke test and Rh immunoglobulin (RhIG).
2. Avoid inserting anything into the patient's vagina if placenta previa is suspected. The speculum and/or examination fingers may tear the placenta and exacerbate the bleeding.

PLACENTAL ABRUPTION

What is it?
Premature separation of the placenta from the uterine wall, resulting in internal hemorrhage

What is the incidence?
0.5%–1.5 %

What are risk factors for placental abruption?
Maternal hypertension, trauma, cocaine or tobacco use, preterm premature rupture of membranes, short umbilical cord, polyhydramnios, previous abruption

What are the classic signs and symptoms of placental abruption?
Patient presents with *painful* vaginal bleeding. Blood is a deep-red color ("port wine"), and the patient has uterine tenderness to palpation.

What less common presentations are important to remember?
Twenty percent of abruptions are concealed (i.e., no vaginal bleeding), and abdominal pain with uterine tenderness is the only finding. Rarely, the patient has neither pain nor significant tenderness.

What diagnostic tests are used?
As with any third-trimester bleeding, CBC with platelets, liver function tests, and clotting studies are indicated. Ultrasound is not reliable in detecting abruption but is performed to rule out placenta previa. Therefore, placental abruption is frequently diagnosed based on clinical findings.

What are the complications of placental abruption?
DIC: placental abruption is the most common cause of DIC in pregnancy

(20% of abruptions are associated with DIC, often with massive hemorrhage or fetal death)
Fetal death: 35% perinatal mortality
Maternal death from exsanguination

How is abruption treated?

Deliver fetus as soon as possible (vaginally, if possible).
Monitor for excessive blood loss and DIC carefully by following coagulation studies and hematocrit closely.

UTERINE RUPTURE

What is it?

A tear through the entire thickness of the uterine wall

What is the incidence of uterine rupture?

0.5%

What are the risk factors for uterine rupture?

1. **Uterine scar** from previous caesarean section or other surgery (40% of ruptures):
   With a previous low transverse caesarean section, the risk is 0.5%.
   With a previous classic vertical caesarean section, the risk is 5%.
2. **Other risk factors** (60% of ruptures):
   Use of oxytocin
   Grand multiparity
   Abnormal fetal lie
   Cephalopelvic disproportion
   External version
   Midforceps delivery
   Trauma

What are the signs and symptoms of uterine rupture?

Intense pain with rupture, followed by a pain-free period, then return of pain. Uterus and abdomen may be tender to palpation. Manual exploration after delivery of infant can detect rupture.

What diagnostic tests are used?

There are no laboratory or radiologic tests that can reliably diagnose uterine rupture.

How is uterine rupture treated if it is detected prior to delivery?	Immediate operative delivery (caesarean section) with repair of uterus, if possible. If repair is not possible, hysterectomy is required.
How is uterine rupture treated if it is detected after delivery?	Large defects require surgical repair or hysterectomy. The best method for treating small defects is less clear. Although most would surgically repair all small defects, there is indirect evidence that they may close without treatment.
Helpful hints	Manual exploration of the uterus after all vaginal deliveries in patients with previous caesarean section is recommended by some physicians, but this practice is not supported by available evidence from clinical trials.

FETAL BLEEDING

What is it?	Vaginal bleeding from a fetal source
What is the incidence?	0.1%–0.8%
What is the most common cause?	Velamentous cord insertion to the placenta
How common is a velamentous cord insertion?	It is found in 1% of single pregnancies, 10% of twin pregnancies, and 50% of triplet pregnancies.
What is the term for velamentous vessels that pass over cervical os?	Vasa previa
What are the signs and symptoms of fetal bleeding?	Vaginal bleeding associated with fetal tachycardia; as the bleeding continues, bradycardia occurs and, as fetal distress worsens, a sinusoidal heart rate pattern occurs
What diagnostic test is used to detect fetal bleeding?	The Apt test detects fetal hemoglobin in vaginal blood.
How is fetal bleeding treated?	Immediate cesarean section

RH DISEASE

What is it?	An incompatibility between maternal and fetal blood antigens. An Rh-positive fetus can sensitize an Rh-negative mother whose immune system makes antibodies to Rh positive. These antibodies can cross the placenta in the same or subsequent pregnancies, causing hemolytic disease of the newborn (erythroblastosis fetalis).
What is Rh?	It is a blood group delineated by an erythrocyte cell membrane protein found on chromosome 1. It is named for the Rhesus monkeys whose erythrocytes, when injected into rabbits, produce antibodies that agglutinated erythrocytes from 85% of Caucasian subjects. There are variations of the Rh antigen gene, of which the antigen D is the most clinically relevant. In addition, a subset of the D variety, known as Du, stimulates anti-D antibodies; therefore, a person who is Rh-negative but Du-positive is considered Rh-positive.
What causes maternal sensitization?	Fetomaternal hemorrhage
How does fetomaternal hemorrhage occur?	At delivery (most common cause) Abdominal trauma Abruption Abortion Amniocentesis Idiopathic
In idiopathic fetomaternal hemorrhage, what percent of pregnancies have detectable fetal cells?	
In the first trimester?	7%
In the second trimester?	16%
In the third trimester?	29%

How is fetomaternal hemorrhage detected?

The Kleihauer-Betke test shows the number of fetal cells in a given volume of maternal blood.

How much blood is needed to sensitize?

Many factors are involved, but as little as 0.1 ml of Rh-positive blood has been shown to sensitize Rh-negative volunteers.

How can it be prevented?

RhIG is used to block fetal cells from sensitizing Rh-negative mothers.

What is the schedule for testing and treating unsensitized pregnant patients with RhIG?

First prenatal visit—Check ABO and Rh status along with antibody screen (indirect Coombs' test).
28 weeks—If patient is Rh-negative, give RhIG.
After delivery—If patient is Rh-negative and infant is Rh-positive or DU positive, give RhIG.

Why is RhIG given at 28 weeks EGA?

Sensitization is rare before 28 weeks. The immunoglobulin persists 12–14 weeks (until term) in most pregnancies.

What is the meaning of a positive antibody screen?

The mother has been previously sensitized to the Rh (or other) antigen, and the fetus is at high risk for complications from these maternal antibodies.

How is RhIG given?

There are 300 μg of anti-D in each vial of RhIG. This vial treats 30 ml of whole Rh-positive blood or 15 ml of packed red blood cells. Usually, one vial is adequate prophylaxis. If concerned about a larger bleed, the Kleihauer-Betke test can quantify how much RhIG is needed.

Helpful hints

1. In patients with first trimester abortions (elective or spontaneous), you must check the patient's blood type; if Rh-negative, administer RhIG.
2. Rh-negative patients who undergo amniocentesis or who have abdominal trauma should receive RhIG.

3. If a patient requires RhIG after 16 weeks EGA (but before 28 weeks EGA), she needs another dose of RhIG 12 weeks after the first dose to ensure adequate RhIG is present at delivery. If RhIG is administered before 16 weeks EGA, the usual dose at 28 weeks is administered per the typical schedule.

HIV DISEASE IN PREGNANCY

What is it?

HIV is a retrovirus that targets T lymphocytes (CD4, or helper T cells) for its replication. The virus eventually destroys the lymphocytes and cripples the immune system. It is acquired by contact with infected body fluids from sexual contact (heterosexual and homosexual), shared needles, contaminated blood or blood products, and vertically from infected mother to infant. This last group represents one of the fastest growing subpopulations victimized by HIV. Although recent developments in treatment are promising, no cure exists.

What is the risk of vertical transmission?

In most studies, between 25%–30%

What factors increase the risk?

Advanced maternal disease (CD4 count
    below 200)
Preterm delivery
Breast feeding

Does cesarean section decrease the risk?

This is a controversial issue. Some studies, but not all, show a slight decrease in transmission.

How can the risk be decreased?

By identifying pregnant women with HIV. The AIDS Clinical Trial Group Protocol 76 gave zidovudine (AZT) to HIV-positive women who had not taken AZT previously, had CD4 counts above 200, and were between 14 and 34 weeks' gestation. They were also given AZT intravenously during labor, and their infants were given AZT postpartum. These patients were compared to similar patients who were administered placebo. The study showed a decrease in transmission from 25% to 8%.

What does this study mean to clinical practice?

All pregnant women should be informed of the advantages of treatment to prevent transmission and strongly encouraged to be tested for HIV.

Are there other treatments available that may help?

A new class of drugs, known as protease inhibitors, when combined with nucleoside analogues like AZT have been shown to reduce HIV virus in the serum to undetectable levels in adults. This is very encouraging, but its application to preventing vertical transmission remains to be seen.

14 Prevention Issues in Primary Care Medicine

What is preventive medicine?

Interventions (e.g., lifestyle changes, medications, tests) aimed at:

Primary prevention: preventing a patient from acquiring a disease

Case finding: finding and treating a disease before it becomes symptomatic or untreatable

Secondary prevention: preventing a recurrence of a previously treated disease

How is preventive medicine different from treating a medical problem?

The contract with the patient changes dramatically. Physicians contract that preventive interventions will make the patient healthier. There is no longer the risk–benefit of therapy versus advancement of illness. Because the patient has neither symptoms nor illness, there is no benefit, only risk of further intervention (unless we have good evidence that our interventions effectively prevent disease). The patient's expectation is that preventive interventions, in the long run, lower medical costs, morbidity, and mortality.

What components of a disease must be present for screening to be effective?

High prevalence: present in a large portion of the population screened

High burden of suffering: causes significant morbidity and/or mortality

Has an asymptomatic stage where detection and effective treatment are possible

Effective treatment is available

Treatment of the asymptomatic stage results in better outcomes than later therapy

What components of a test must be present for screening to be effective?

Accuracy
Safety
Reasonable cost
Acceptability to patients

What burden of evidence must be met before use of a screening strategy is ethical?

The extra cost to the patient in money, time, and effort to undergo the intervention is only justifiable if the benefits and outcomes the patient cares about (e.g., lower cost, morbidity, mortality, time lost from work) are assured. The benefits must be verified in well-designed randomized, controlled clinical trials. Other, less rigorous studies or studies that only look at intermediate outcomes do not adequately meet this ethical standard.

What two factors cause even well-designed screening studies to overestimate the benefit of screening?

Lead-time bias
Length-time bias

What is lead-time bias?

It is a shift in the detection time of a disease because of the screening. When screening for a disease, it is found earlier in its natural history than in the population not being screened (i.e., control group). By finding the disease earlier than usual (i.e., lead time), the screened population appears healthier than the control group, even if screening and intervention do not change the natural history of the disease. This bias occurs because the control group is farther along the course of the disease and appears to have more adverse effects because they have had the disease longer.

What is length-time bias?

It is the tendency of screening to detect persons with a less aggressive form of a disease. Patients with a more aggressive form of the disease tend to die sooner. Therefore, they are less likely to be found by a screening test because they are present in the population for a shorter period of time than persons with less aggressive forms of the disease. The result is that the screening test overestimates the true benefit of the test because fewer people with more aggressive disease are included in the study.

Why is it important to consider all these issues when deciding which preventive interventions to use?

Primary care practitioners are extremely busy and have only a limited amount of time to spend on prevention. Patients, and the health care system as a whole, have limited resources. The community must concentrate preventive efforts and resources on those interventions that have a high likelihood of being successful. Otherwise, resources are wasted.

What tests often done for screening are not indicated for otherwise healthy patients?

Chest radiograph
Electrocardiogram
Exercise stress tests
Multiple test serum chemistry panels

Name some national medical groups that have developed recommendations for periodic screening.

A few examples include:
The American Academy of Family
  Physicians (AAFP)
American College of Physicians (ACP)
American Cancer Society (ACS)
United States Preventive Health Task
  Force (USPHTF)

Which group used a rigorous evidence-based approach in the development of its guidelines?

The USPHTF—their publication, *Guide to Clinical Preventive Services* (Williams & Wilkins, 1995) is a comprehensive summary of data and a good resource for developing preventive strategies.

How does a physician decide which screening tests to perform on a patient?

Screening strategies should be tailored to each patient's individual risk profile. The risk assessment is the key to choosing appropriate screening tests.

What is a risk profile?

It is a comprehensive review of the patient's medical, social, and family history that is used to identify illnesses or problems for which the patient is at high risk.

Why is the risk profile important?	Statistically, all tests have a better positive predictive value in groups with a high prevalence of disease. The risk profile helps stratify the patient into high- or low-prevalence groups. The screening strategy can then be developed to maximize the usefulness of tests (i.e., tests with a better positive predictive based on the prevalence of the disease in patients with similar risk) and other interventions.

CASE EXAMPLES

A 55-year-old overweight woman who smokes and is sedentary has adult-onset diabetes mellitus, hypertension, and a strong family history of ischemic heart disease. She has been married for 30 years, has two children that she breast fed, is in a mutually monogamous relationship, and has 20 years of normal Pap smears (last Pap was one year ago).

What is her risk assessment?	She is at very high risk for coronary artery disease, increased risk for osteoporosis, average risk for breast cancer, and very low risk for cervical cancer.
What screening tests should be ordered?	Cholesterol, mammography; consider exercise stress test before exercise prescription
What screening test is not indicated?	Pap smear
What interventions are indicated?	Smoking cessation, blood pressure control, low-fat diet, exercise prescription, hormone replacement, and calcium supplementation.

A 25 year-old-woman does not smoke, exercises regularly, and has no family history of heart disease or breast cancer. She has had six sexual partners in the past year; only occasionally have her partners used condoms. She has previous mild abnormalities on Pap smear.

What is her risk assessment?	She is at high risk for cervical cancer and STDs. She is at low risk for breast cancer (due to her age) and very low risk for coronary artery disease.

What screening tests should be ordered?	Pap smear; consider gonorrhea and chlamydia cultures and HIV testing
What screening tests are not indicated?	Cholesterol testing, mammography
What interventions are indicated?	Counsel about changing high-risk sexual activity
Helpful hints	Avoid a "cookbook" approach to prevention. Remain wary of recommendations developed by consensus panels. (See Chapter 18, Evidenced-Based Medicine.)

15   Common Psychiatric Problems

ATTENTION DEFICIT HYPERACTIVITY DISORDER (ADHD) / ATTENTION DEFICIT DISORDER WITHOUT HYPERACTIVITY (ADD)

What is it?

A clinical syndrome manifested by an individual's inability to maintain concentration on a task or inability to remain still long enough to complete a task. The deficit must significantly interfere with the patient's performance (social, school, or work) and be inappropriate for age and development.

What causes it?

There are many theories that attempt to explain ADHD/ADD, but the cause is unknown. It is most likely a common clinical pathway with multiple etiologies.

What is the prevalence of ADHD in school-age children?

$2\% - 4\%$

What is the male to female ratio for prevalence of ADHD?

$3:1$

Do ADHD and ADD only occur in childhood?

No. It is estimated that up to 60% of children with these disorders will have symptoms that persist into adulthood.

What are the common symptoms of ADHD/ADD?

Poor school performance
Behavior problems
Activity levels well above those expected for age
Impulsive behaviors (performing acts without considering risk or danger)
Distractibility
Poor peer interactions

What are some of the other problems that can cause similar symptoms?	Learning disabilities Visual acuity problems Hearing problems Psychosocial stress (e.g., abuse, neglect, family problems) Depression Oppositional – Defiant Disorder Conduct Disorder Mental retardation Organic brain syndromes (e.g., lead poisoning) Hyperthyroidism
What is found on physical examination of patients with ADHD/ADD?	The patient usually tries very hard to cooperate but has difficulty maintaining focus. Sometimes, subtle abnormalities can be found on neurologic examination, but in most cases the examination findings are normal.
What should be included in an evaluation of a patient with suspected ADHD/ADD?	This is controversial. Some clinicians initiate treatment with just a brief history from the teacher or parent; this approach often leads to overtreatment and can miss potentially important behavioral or learning problems. A more conservative approach is to evaluate for visual and hearing deficits and metabolic problems; if no abnormalities are found, a full evaluation of the patient's learning, cognitive, and behavioral abilities is undertaken. Standardized questionnaires can be administered to parents and teachers to help confirm the diagnosis and give a baseline from which treatment can be measured.
How are ADHD and ADD treated?	Behavioral management Parenting skills augmentation Medication
What types of medications are used to treat ADHD/ADD?	**Stimulants:** methylphenidate, dextroamphetamine, pemoline **Antidepressants:** desipramine, imipramine, bupropion, fluoxetine
What class of medication is used most frequently?	Stimulants

How often will stimulant medication be effective?	60% – 80% of patients will benefit.
What are the most common side effects of stimulant therapy?	Decreased appetite; may lead to poor growth or weight loss Insomnia Abdominal pain Headache Lethargy Irritability Mild hypertension or tachycardia
How can these side effects be avoided?	Using the lowest effective dose Drug holidays (such as on weekends and other days off from school or work)
How can the strong placebo effect of medication (for the patient, parents, and teachers) be evaluated?	By performing a placebo-controlled trial when therapy is initiated
How is this accomplished?	The pharmacist prepares four bottles of medication for the 4-week trial: two with active medication and two with placebo. The pharmacist decides the order in which the bottles are to be used and instructs the parents, but does not reveal which bottles contain placebo and which contain active medication. The parents and teachers complete a standardized evaluation form at the end of each week; the evaluation forms are graded by the physician. The scores are then reviewed at the end of the 4-week period and compared with the treatment/placebo schedule set up by the pharmacist. Significant improvement should be evident on parental and teacher scales during weeks with active medication to confirm treatment benefit.
Helpful hints:	1. There is often a great deal of pressure placed on the physician to give stimulants to children with behavioral problems or poor school performance. Insist on appropriate evaluation and behavioral

interventions before initiating medication.

2. Children with ADHD or ADD are at high risk for abuse because of the many challenges they present to the parents.

3. Children with ADHD or ADD are at high risk for depression and substance abuse, both from the nature of the problem and from low self-esteem issues.

ANXIETY DISORDERS

What are they?

A group of clinical syndromes with a wide spectrum of manifestations whose common symptoms are nervousness or fear that causes social or physical dysfunction

Is anxiety always dysfunctional?

No. In most situations, anxiety motivates us to attend to problems or change the environment in some way to eliminate the stimulus causing the anxiety.

In what ways are persons with anxiety disorders dysfunctional?

The anxiety is so overwhelming that their social functioning is impaired, their life processes are impaired (e.g., sleep), or their health is affected.

What are common causes of anxiety disorders?

Previous emotional trauma (e.g., death of loved one, abuse), psychosocial stress, irrational thought processes (e.g., agoraphobia), or impaired coping skills

What are some of the most common anxiety disorders?

Generalized Anxiety Disorder
Adjustment Disorder
Phobias
Panic Attacks

What are common symptoms of persons with anxiety disorders?

Nervousness, fear, insomnia, palpitations, numbness or tingling, nausea, diarrhea, constipation, headache, chest pain, abdominal pain, back pain, hypochondriasis, and depressed mood. Certain situations (e.g., crowded areas, leaving the house) may precipitate symptoms.

What are the common physical findings in patients with anxiety?

Tachycardia, tachypnea, and elevated blood pressure may be found. The physical examination usually reveals little else that is helpful in making the diagnosis.

What tests are indicated in patients with anxiety disorders?

- Using one of the many questionnaires validated to measure anxiety can help with diagnosis or evaluation of treatment.
- Consider evaluation of thyroid function and other hypermetabolic states if indicated by history or physical examination findings.
- Formal psychiatric testing should be considered if symptoms are atypical or recalcitrant to treatment.

How are anxiety disorders treated?

Cognitive therapy
Biofeedback
Medication

What are the most common medications used to treat anxiety disorders?

Buspirone
Benzodiazepines
Selective serotonin reuptake inhibitors (SSRIs)

What are the admission criteria?

Persons with significant risk for suicide should be admitted (with court order, if necessary) and observed closely in an appropriate environment.

Helpful hints:

1. Persons with acute anxiety syndromes (i.e., panic attacks) are at increased risk for suicide and should be evaluated for this risk.
2. *Overprescribing of benzodiazepines is still a major problem. These agents are highly addictive; they should be used with caution and only in patients with appropriate diagnoses.*
3. Anxiety frequently accompanies depression. Patients should be evaluated for depression before therapy for anxiety is initiated.

MAJOR DEPRESSION

What is it?	A mood disorder that impairs the ability to interact with the environment in a positive way and is accompanied by changes in physiologic processes
What causes it?	The current theory is that certain neurotransmitters in the brain (serotonin and dopamine) become altered in concentration or function. These alterations are thought to cause both the behavioral and physiologic symptoms.
How common is depression?	Up to 85% of people will have a major depressive episode in their lifetimes.
What are the common behavioral symptoms of depression?	Depressed mood Decreased libido Anhedonia (inability to experience happiness) Hopelessness Crying spells Irritability Poor concentration Anxiety Suicidal ideation
What are the common physiologic symptoms of depression?	Insomnia Change in appetite Fatigue Psychomotor slowing
What is the pattern of insomnia in depression?	The sleep latency (time needed to fall asleep) is normal. The patient will awaken early in the morning hours and not be able to fall back to sleep, often for several hours.
What are common physical findings in patients with depression?	Flat affect and slow thought processes are hallmarks of depression. The physical examination findings are usually otherwise normal.
What issue must be carefully explored in each patient with depression before outpatient treatment is initiated?	Suicide risk

Should every patient with suicidal thoughts be hospitalized?

No; suicidal thoughts are common. However, if the patient has developed a plan for suicide, or acquired the means to carry out a plan, strong consideration must be given to admission (by court order, if necessary) and close observation.

What diagnostic tests are used for depression?

Questionnaires have been developed to evaluate the likelihood of depression; they can also be helpful in evaluating treatment. Formal psychological testing (e.g., the Minnesota Multiphasic Personality Inventory) can be used in patients with atypical symptoms. Since thyroid disease is fairly common and can have symptoms similar to those of depression, obtaining a TSH level should be considered in each patient before treatment is initiated. Most of the time, however, treatment is initiated without further tests (i.e., with a history and physical examination findings consistent with the diagnosis).

How is depression treated?

Cognitive therapy and counseling
Medication

What is the most effective treatment approach?

A combination of cognitive therapy and medication is better than either approach used alone.

What classes of medications are used to treat depression?

Tricyclic antidepressants (TCAs)—for example, imipramine, amitriptyline
SSRIs—for example, fluoxetine, sertraline
Monoamine oxidase inhibitors (MAOs)
Others—nefazodone, bupropion

Is one class more effective than another?

No; all are equally effective.

What are the differences between classes?

Price
Side effects
Interactions with other drugs or foods

What are common adverse effects of each class?

TCAs—drowsiness, dry mucous membranes, weight gain, urinary

retention, constipation, postural hypotension, cardiac arrhythmias in excessive doses or overdose

SSRIs—agitation, nausea, anorexia, sexual dysfunction; expensive

MAOs—risk of interaction with multiple drugs and foods, resulting in marked hypertension with potential cardiac and CNS complications

Others—unique to each agent (Lowering the seizure threshold is of concern for with some of these agents.)

Which class of drugs is seldom used by primary care physicians, and why?

MAOs, because the increased risk of harmful side effects limits their use to refractory cases that generally require specialty input

Are SSRIs better tolerated than TCAs?

Despite many claims that SSRIs are better tolerated than TCAs, there is no evidence to support this claim. Randomized controlled trials comparing agents from both classes showed no difference in pooled dropout rates (i.e., patients discontinuing the drug because they could not tolerate it). This would indicate that the side effects of the SSRIs, while different, are no better tolerated than those of the TCAs.

What are the admission criteria?

1. Patients with a significant risk for suicide
2. Patients with psychotic features to their depression

Helpful hints:

1. Many persons with substance abuse problems are "self-medicating" for depression. Therefore, screening substance-abusing patients for depression is an important part of their evaluation.
2. Families of depressed patients often need support and education in order to understand how this disease affects their loved ones.
3. *Patients with suicidal ideation must be monitored closely after therapy is initiated.* Psychomotor slowing may

improve before the depressed mood, providing these patients with the energy to act on their suicidal ideations.

SUBSTANCE ABUSE

What is it?

A clinical syndrome characterized by the continued use of any substance despite negative physical, social, or legal consequences

What is the magnitude of the problem?

- More people die in the United States each year from illness related to tobacco use than from any other single cause.
- One fourth of adults use tobacco products.
- Medical costs of consequences of substance abuse are staggering.
- Eight to ten million Americans have problems with alcohol abuse.
- Law enforcement related to alcohol and tobacco sales and illegal drug traffic costs billions of dollars each year.

What are some of the common physical consequences of substance abuse?

Major and minor trauma
Sexually transmitted diseases
Infertility
Impotence
Diseases (including cancer) of the heart, liver, lung, pancreas, or GI tract

What are some of the common social and legal consequences encountered by substance abusers?

Relationship difficulties (with spouse, children, parents, siblings, friends)
Employment difficulties
Arrests for driving under the influence of alcohol
Arrests for possession of illegal drugs
Arrests for violent behaviors
High-risk sexual behaviors (e.g., promiscuity, not using barrier protection for STDs)

Does substance abuse always involve substance dependence (addiction)?

No; the two often coexist, but abuse behaviors do not always include addiction.

What are the two most common drugs of abuse?	Nicotine (tobacco products) Alcohol
What are some other common drugs of abuse?	Opioids Cocaine Cannabis (marijuana) Benzodiazepines Phencyclidine (PCP) Hallucinogens (e.g., LSD)
What are risk factors for substance abuse?	Family history of substance abuse Personal history of substance abuse Victim of family violence/abuse Persons with other psychiatric diagnoses (e.g., depression, anxiety)
Are all persons who use substances of abuse substance abusers? Explain.	No; there appears to be a continuum of use patterns. This continuum begins at abstinence and progresses through occasional use and misuse to abuse and addiction. Some persons are able to use these substances and avoid the abuse/addiction end of the spectrum.
How can we identify persons with substance abuse problems?	Ask. All patients should be questioned regularly about their use of tobacco, alcohol, and other drugs. Patients who give positive responses should be asked follow-up questions to evaluate the extent of the problem. Questionnaires (such as the CAGE questions) can be helpful in distinguishing use from abuse. Studies suggest that physicians can have a positive impact on persons with risky use patterns, but frequently don't ask their patients about potential substance problems.
What is the major stumbling block to treatment?	Denial. Most persons with substance abuse problems do not identify themselves as having a problem. Participation of family, friends, or employers may assist with getting the substance abuser into treatment.
What issues need to be addressed in treatment of substance abuse?	**Medical**—Treat withdrawal symptoms or metabolic complications of withdrawal (these will vary from substance to substance).

Psychological—There are often many issues that need addressing. Referral for counseling services can be very helpful. Identification and treatment of coexisting psychiatric problems (e.g., depression, anxiety disorders) can increase success of interventions for substance abuse.

Social—Family and work relationships are usually impaired; these problems are often what motivates the substance abuser to seek treatment. The family will need support and counseling to deal with the many issues involved with substance abuse, treatment, and aftercare.

How can I, as a health-care provider, be more effective in helping persons with substance abuse problems?

Be direct. Directly address your concerns with the patient. Review the potential medical consequences of the patient's behavior. Point out social and legal consequences, if they exist. Refute efforts by the patient to deny the problem.

Show support. Remember that substance abuse is a medical problem. Patients already often have low self-esteem, so avoid actions or statements that could be interpreted as judgmental. Patients are much more likely to respond positively to expressions of genuine concern. Changing substance abuse behaviors is a long process, and the patient needs your help long-term. There is a fine line between support and enabling, so carefully consider the long-term consequence of each decision.

Be persistent. Review your concerns with the patient during each visit and give positive reinforcement for progress. It takes most people some time to change their behavior. There will usually be relapses even in motivated patients.

Identify enablers. The substance abuser often has a family member with a co-dependent personality. The co-dependent person enables the substance abuser to continue to use the substance by dealing with the negative consequences of the abuser's actions (e.g., lying to an employer that a spouse is sick when he or she is really drunk). Convincing the enabler to cease enabling behaviors will help the substance abuser experience directly the consequences of his or her actions and, hopefully, provide impetus for treatment. Once again, avoid being an enabler yourself.

What community resources are available to help patients deal with substance abuse?

Substance abuse treatment programs assist the patient at the beginning of the treatment program. They often assist with the patient's withdrawal from addictive substances and provide structure during a very chaotic time for the patient.

Support groups provide a supportive environment and peer feedback, and decrease the isolation the patient feels as he or she radically changes. Examples are Alcoholics Anonymous (AA) and smoking cessation support groups.

Family support groups help families of substance abusers cope with the consequences of living with (or having previously lived with) a substance abuser and help them learn to avoid enabling behaviors. Examples are Al-Anon and Al-Ateen.

What are the admission criteria?

1. Patients withdrawing from substances with potentially serious withdrawal syndromes (e.g., alcohol, barbiturates) and patients with previous history of serious medical complications during drug withdrawal (e.g., seizures, delirium tremens) should be admitted for detoxification.

2. Substance abusers are at high risk for perpetrating family violence or abuse; this potential should be investigated in all cases of substance abuse.

Helpful hints:

1. Patients with substance abuse problems often have other psychiatric problems and high levels of psychosocial stress. Addressing or treating these associated conditions may help the patient have more success dealing with the substance abuse.
2. If possible, avoid prescribing potentially addicting drugs to patients with active or previous substance abuse problems. If it is unavoidable, monitor use closely.
3. Many people become addicted to prescription drugs each year. Use of potentially addictive agents should be limited to appropriate indications and monitored closely.

FAMILY VIOLENCE/ABUSE/NEGLECT (V/A/N)

What are they?

A wide spectrum of dysfunctional behaviors that range from inadequately caring for a dependent family member at one end of the spectrum, to homicide at the other. Degrading verbal abuse, physical abuse, and sexual abuse are other dysfunctional behaviors included in the V/A/N spectrum.

What risk factors help identify potential perpetrators of V/A/N?

Witnessed or was a victim of family violence/abuse/neglect as a child
Substance abuse
Psychological or personality disorder
Male gender
High level of psychosocial stress

What are some of the signs and symptoms of victims of V/A/N?

Failure to thrive (child or adult)
Violent behaviors exhibited at school or in the office
Somatization
Hypochondriasis
Anxiety
Depression (especially in a child)
Encopresis
Secondary enuresis
Traumatic injuries (especially recurrent injuries) inconsistent with the

mechanism of injury described by the caretaker (e.g., fractured humerus in a child who "fell down while running on the lawn")

Children with recurrent unexplained illnesses

What is the primary responsibility of the physician in cases of V/A/N?

The safety of the at-risk family member(s) should be the primary concern.

How is this addressed for children?

Laws vary from state to state, but most states have statutes requiring health-care professionals to report suspected cases of V/A/N to a social service agency for investigation. Most states also give the physician the option of admitting the child for observation for a short period of time (even against the wishes of the parents or guardians) in situations deemed imminently dangerous for the child; the concern is investigated by social services while the child is protected.

How is this addressed for adults?

Dependent adults (frail, elderly family members who cannot care for themselves) require an approach similar to the one for children, with notification of social services mandated in most states.

Independent adults (usually women) are provided with or encouraged to use shelters or to seek protection from law enforcement officials. Fear of violent reprisals from the perpetrator and issues of codependency can delay victims from availing themselves of these resources. Close follow-up and support are essential for monitoring the patient's well-being and for continuing efforts to encourage the patient to move to a safe environment.

After all at-risk family members are safe, what is the role of the physician?

Appropriate referrals so that the victims can receive psychological support and counseling

Intervention with perpetrators so that they can receive appropriate help

What are the admission criteria?

1. Physical injuries requiring hospital care
2. The need for temporary protection in situations of imminent danger for children and dependent adults (i.e., dependent family member may be subjected to additional abuse if returned to family situation)

Helpful hints:

1. Carefully document all physical findings of suspected victims of V/A/N.
2. Be sure to avoid leading questions with children. (Ask, "What happened to cause this?" Not, "Did your daddy do this to you?")
3. Families with documented V/A/N are at high risk for recurrent problems, even with appropriate intervention.

16   Common Respiratory Problems

ASTHMA

What is it?	A type of reactive airways disease characterized by an inflammatory reaction in the bronchioles of the lung, which results in contraction of bronchial smooth muscle and overproduction of endobronchial mucus secondary to a number of stimuli
What are some of the common stimuli (triggers) for asthma?	Allergens—pollen, mold, dust mites Irritants—smoke, dust, dry air Respiratory tract infections Exercise (usually occurs 10–20 minutes after beginning exercise) Circadian rhythm (Evening or nighttime can be associated with symptoms.) Air temperature (Cold air is more often a trigger than warm air.) Idiopathic (no specific stimulus identified) Aspiration—secondary to GERD (see Chapter 8)
What is the cardinal sign/symptom of asthma?	Wheezing
What is wheezing?	Wheezing is a high-pitched whistling sound usually heard on expiration during auscultation of the lungs, but sometimes during inspiration. Wheezing may also be heard without the stethoscope, which is why it is both a symptom and a sign of asthma.
What are other common symptoms of asthma?	Dyspnea Cough Chest tightness

What are other common signs of asthma?	Tachypnea Tachycardia Retractions (supraclavicular, intercostal, subdiaphragmatic) Hypoxia *As the patient fatigues:* cyanosis, absent breath sounds, and hypercarbia
What are common tests used in the outpatient evaluation of patients with asthma?	Peak flow measurement Percutaneous measurement of oxygen saturation of hemoglobin (O_2 sat)
How is the peak flow measurement used to monitor asthma?	The peak flow is initially measured when the patient is doing well. When the patient is having symptoms, treatment decisions are made using the percent reduction in peak flow from baseline.
How is asthma treated?	Inhaled bronchodilators—short-acting β-agonists (albuterol, terbutaline, etc.) and long-acting β-agonists (salmeterol) Inhaled anti-inflammatory agents—corticosteroids and mast cell stabilizers (cromolyn, nedocromil) Inhaled anticholinergic agent—ipratropium Systemic selective leukotriene receptor antagonist (oral)—zafirlukast Systemic corticosteroids (oral or parenteral) Systemic theophylline preparations (oral or parenteral)
How are inhaled bronchodilators used in the treatment of asthma?	They are used as needed (p.r.n.) to control symptoms, up to every 3–4 hours. Persons with exercise-induced asthma use the medication 15–20 minutes before exercise. If the patient is using the medication more than 1–2 times each week, anti-inflammatory agents should be considered.
How are anti-inflammatory agents used in the treatment of asthma?	They are used on a regular schedule. The goal is for the medication to block the initiation of the inflammatory process that leads to asthma symptoms.

Frequent use of β-agonists indicates a chronic process that can often be interrupted by an anti-inflammatory agent.

What is the current role of theophylline in the treatment of asthma?

Theophylline was once a first-line agent; now it is used only when the other treatments fail, or when there are significant nighttime symptoms that occur between doses of β-agonists and that are not controlled with anti-inflammatory agents.

What is the rationale for using inhaled medication?

The medication is delivered directly to the location where it is needed (the bronchioles). Systemic side effects can be avoided or minimized.

What is the most common method for administering inhaled medication?

Metered dose inhalers (MDIs)

Why should spacing devices be used with MDIs?

They allow more medication to be delivered to the bronchioles.

How is this accomplished by a spacer?

1. It eliminates the need for the exact coordination of inspiration with activation of the MDI.
2. It allows for deceleration of the medication before inhalation. This decreases the amount of medication that impacts and adheres to the mucous membranes of the mouth and pharynx.

What is the other device used to deliver inhaled medication?

The nebulizer

Is the nebulizer better than the MDI (with spacer) at administering inhaled medication?

No. If enough puffs from the MDI are used to equal the dose of medication administered by the nebulizer, they are equally effective at delivering the medication, and the clinical response of the patient is the same. However, some patients find it easier to get higher doses of inhaled medications through the nebulizer.

Which category of medication administered by MDI is *not* given by nebulizer?

Corticosteroids

When treating asthma, are corticosteroids administered intravenously more effective than those administered by mouth?

No. The time to onset and magnitude of response are the same regardless of route of administration.

How can treatment options and clinical information be combined into an organized approach to patients with asthma?

1. Begin with a short-acting β-agonist; use as a single agent for infrequent or exercise-induced asthma. Continue use and increase dose or frequency, or both, as level of severity worsens.
2. Add inhaled anti-inflammatory agents early. Anyone with frequent or regular symptoms, or acute episodes with a decrease in peak flow of 20% to 40% below baseline, would benefit from these agents.
3. Add inhaled anticholinergics if symptoms are not controlled with inhaled anti-inflammatory agents.
4. Add zafirlukast if symptoms are not controlled with inhaled anti-inflammatory agents.
5. Add systemic corticosteroids for brief periods if acute symptoms are associated with a decrease in peak flow of greater than 40%, or if acute symptoms do not readily abate with increased doses of β-agonists. Avoid long-term systemic corticosteroids.
6. Salmeterol and theophylline are usually reserved for persistent nocturnal symptoms that do not respond to other measures.

What are the admission criteria?

1. Status asthmaticus (see below)
2. Any level of respiratory compromise in a patient with new-onset disease, unfamiliar with use of medications, or not in a position to quickly access the health-care system (i.e., no phone, no assistance at home, lives far from the hospital)

Helpful hints:

1. Desensitization therapy (allergy shots) has not been shown to change the frequency or severity of asthma in patients with allergic components to their disease.
2. Do not assume that all patients with wheezing have asthma. Many other disease processes can cause wheezing.
3. Chest x-ray (CXR) is not indicated in patients with an acute exacerbation of asthma unless signs and symptoms of lower respiratory tract infection are also present.

STATUS ASTHMATICUS

What is it?

Persistence of severe asthma symptoms despite therapy. It is a medical emergency because it can lead to respiratory failure and death.

What are signs and symptoms of status asthmaticus?

The same as asthma, but more severe. In addition, fatigue, cyanosis, and marked retractions with use of accessory muscles of respiration (e.g., sternomastoid, trapezius) can occur. Fatigue and failure of respiratory muscles can lead to respiratory failure, apnea, and death.

What tests are used in patients with status asthmaticus?

O_2 sat
Arterial blood gases (ABGs)
CXR

What changes in the ABGs indicate impending problems?

Problems are indicated when the ABGs shift from the initial respiratory alkalosis (from hyperventilation) with mild hypoxia of moderate asthma, to a normal or low pH with a trend of increasing P_{CO_2} and decreasing P_{O_2}. These changes reflect increasing fatigue of respiratory muscles and impending respiratory failure.

How is status asthmaticus treated?

• Aggressive use of inhaled β-agonists—Frequency is increased as needed until the administration of continuous nebulized β-agonist can be used, if necessary.

- High-dose systemic corticosteroids—These are usually administered intravenously because of the severity of the illness.
- Ipratropium or theophylline, or both, can be used for patients who don't respond quickly to therapy.
- Close monitoring with continuous O_2 sats, frequent vital signs, and frequent or continuous nebulizer treatments may necessitate admission to an intensive care unit.
- Endotracheal intubation with mechanical ventilation may be needed.

ALLERGIC RHINITIS

What is it?
Rhinitis caused by an allergic response in the upper respiratory tract

What are common allergens that cause allergic rhinitis?
Pollens
Dust mites
Animal danders
Molds

What is the main risk factor?
Family history of atopic diseases (asthma, allergic rhinitis, eczema)

What historical factor indicates allergic rhinitis secondary to pollen?
Seasonal variations in symptoms—that is, symptoms occur during the seasons when the pollens are present (e.g., fall for ragweed, early spring for trees)

What are common symptoms of allergic rhinitis?
Itching (eyes, ears, nose, throat)
Watery discharge from the nose or eyes
Sneezing
Nasal congestion

What are common physical findings in patients with allergic rhinitis?
Prominence of blood vessels in the bulbar and palpebral conjunctiva (conjunctival infection)
Dark discoloration of the lower eyelids
Pale/edematous nasal mucosa
Watery nasal discharge
Patchy areas of erythema in the oropharynx

What diagnostic tests can be used in patients with allergic rhinitis?

Serum IgE levels

Total eosinophil count

Swab of nasal secretions stained to identify eosinophils

Tests to identify specific offending allergens (skin tests, serum RAS tests)

How is allergic rhinitis treated?

Antihistamines—sedating side effects frequent with some (diphenhydramine, cetirizine, etc.); others are non-sedating (loratadine, fexofenadine, etc.).

Corticosteroids—intranasal administration by aqueous or non-aqueous formulations

Desensitization—repeated injections with low concentrations of the offending allergen

Avoidance—use of plastic covers for mattress and pillows; minimizing wall-to-wall carpet to avoid dust mites; avoidance of pets with offending danders

Helpful hints:

1. Desensitization is more effective for pollens than for dust mites or molds. It also has the potential side effect of anaphylaxis.
2. Older non-sedating antihistamines (terfenadine, astemizole) have potential drug interactions and adverse effects, and should be avoided.

ACUTE BRONCHITIS (BRONCHITIS)

What is it?

An acute infection of the airways of the lung (bronchi, bronchioles)

What causes the infection?

Viruses

Bacteria—*Streptococcus pneumoniae*, group A streptococcus, *Haemophilus influenzae*

Mycoplasma species

Chlamydia species

Which are the most common cause of bronchitis?	Viruses, by far
What are common signs and symptoms of bronchitis?	Cough Fever Sputum production Wheezing Rhonchi
What diagnostic tests are used?	There are no specific tests to diagnose bronchitis. CXR can exclude pneumonia, and peak flow testing can exclude asthma. Sputum cultures are not helpful.
How is bronchitis treated?	Antitussives Bronchodilators Antibiotics
What is the best medication to decrease symptoms in patients with bronchitis?	Inhaled β-agonists
What are the most common antibiotics used to treat bronchitis?	Amoxicillin Erythromycin Trimethoprim/sulfamethoxazole
Why?	They are effective against the most common bacteria that cause bronchitis.
Helpful hints:	1. Frequently there is a concurrent upper respiratory infection. 2. Smokers with bronchitis are much more likely to benefit from treatment with antibiotics. 3. Codeine is no more effective than dextromethorphan in suppressing cough; they are equally ineffective when compared to inhaled β-agonists.

VIRAL UPPER RESPIRATORY INFECTION (URI)

What is it?	The term "URI" is used for a variety of illnesses that involve viral infections of any portion of the upper respiratory tract—in other words, the common cold.

What are some of the viruses that cause URIs?

Rhinovirus (most common)
  Influenza virus
Parainfluenza virus
Adenovirus
Respiratory syncytial virus

What are the common signs and symptoms of URIs?

Nasal congestion
Nasal discharge
Throat pain
Nonproductive cough
Erythema of the nasal mucosa and
  pharynx
Mild lymphadenopathy
Low-grade fever
Headache

What tests are used to diagnose URI?

None are used; the diagnosis is made clinically. Throat culture and sinus radiographs may sometimes be helpful if there is reason to suspect another infection with similar symptoms (e.g., strep pharyngitis or sinusitis).

What is the main challenge in diagnosing a URI?

Attempting to distinguish the viral infections from the bacterial infections (e.g., group A streptococcal, pharyngitis, bacterial sinusitis) that may require antibiotic therapy

How are URIs treated?

Zinc lozenges have been shown to decrease the duration and intensity of symptoms. Otherwise, symptomatic treatment is used (antipyretics, analgesics, nasal decongestants).

What is the major public health issue related to URI treatment?

Antibiotic-resistant bacteria

Why?

Since the beginning of the antibiotic era, physicians have often treated viral URIs with antibiotics on the outside chance that the infection was bacterial. Over time, many patients came to expect antibiotic therapy for any upper respiratory illness. This combination of physician practice and patient expectation led to the massive overuse of antibiotics. With repeated exposures to antibiotics, bacteria have developed resistance. Even bacteria that had remained susceptible to frequently used antibiotics have now begun to show resistance (e.g., penicillin-resistant streptococci). Resistance makes therapy much more difficult and costly. Some experts espouse the position that it is only a matter of time until widespread resistance will make antibiotics ineffective against almost all bacteria.

How can this problem be improved?

- Limit use of antibiotics to the few diseases for which they have been shown to be effective.
- Use the antibiotic with the most narrow spectrum that will treat the disease.
- Avoid prolonged or repeated administration of antibiotics.

STREPTOCOCCAL PHARYNGITIS (STREP THROAT)

What is it?

A bacterial infection of the pharynx

What causes it?

Group A β-hemolytic streptococci (GABHS)

In a patient with throat pain, what are the four primary signs and symptoms associated with GABHS pharyngitis?

Fever
Lack of cough
Tender anterior cervical lymphadenopathy
Exudative pharyngitis (exudates visualized on the tonsils or pharynx)

What tests are used to diagnose GABHS pharyngitis?

Throat culture (gold standard)
Streptococcus antigen detection tests

What is the limitation of each test?

- Throat cultures take up to 48 hours to give a positive result, so treatment may be delayed, or antibiotics may be given for 48 hours unnecessarily.
- Antigen tests take only a few minutes but have a low specificity, which can lead to missing the presence of GABHS.

How is GABHS pharyngitis treated?	Penicillin VK, 500 mg b.i.d. for 10 days (adults and children over 12 years) Penicillin VK, 250 mg b.i.d. for 10 days (children under 12 years) Erythromycin is used for penicillin-allergic patients.
Does treatment alter the course of the illness?	Unless antibiotics are started in the first 24 hours of the illness, there is no effect on the course of the illness.
Then why is treatment important?	In older children and young adults, untreated GABHS pharyngitis is associated with the development of rheumatic fever.
Helpful hints:	Most physicians use throat culture to diagnose GABHS pharyngitis. However, a rational approach to diagnosis of GABHS pharyngitis using only the antigen test has been proposed by Slawson and co-authors in a letter in *Journal of Family Practice* 39(5):428, 1994 (Nov).

SINUSITIS

What is it?	Sinusitis is an inflammation of any of the paranasal sinuses. Most often, the inflammation is secondary to an infection.
What causes it?	Two conditions usually need to be present for the development of sinusitis: 1. Infecting organisms 2. Impaired drainage secondary to ostial obstruction
What are common organisms that cause sinusitis?	Viruses Bacteria—group A streptococci, *Streptococcus pneumoniae, Haemophilus influenzae, Moraxella catarrhalis, Staphylococcus aureus*
What are the common signs and symptoms of sinusitis?	Nasal congestion and discharge Face pain Pain in the upper teeth Fever Purulent drainage observed from the sinus ostia

Tenderness over the cheeks or frontal areas of the face

Asymmetry with transillumination

What tests are used to diagnose sinusitis?

Usually, treatment is initiated based on signs and symptoms. However, in recurrent or refractory cases or when the diagnosis is unclear, imaging of the paranasal sinuses is considered. Plain x-rays have traditionally been the first choice of imaging modality, but CT scan is more sensitive and is now similar in cost to plain x-rays in many institutions.

How is sinusitis treated?

Reduction or elimination of ostial obstruction

Antibiotics (for bacterial infection)

Surgical drainage

What are first- and second-line antibiotics for sinusitis?

First line—amoxicillin, trimethoprim/ sulfamethoxazole

Second line—amoxicillin/clavulanate, second-generation cephalosporins, clarithromycin

How long should antibiotics be used to treat sinusitis?

Treatment for 14 days is the most frequent recommendation. Double-strength trimethoprim/sulfamethoxazole taken for 3 days has been shown to be effective in 75% of cases of sinusitis; this is a very cost-effective approach, but arrangements must be made to continue treatment for the full 14 days in the 25% who do not respond to the 3-day treatment [Williams JW Jr, et al. Randomized controlled trial of 3 vs. 10 days of trimethoprim/sulfametoxazole for acute maxillary sinusitis. *JAMA* 273(13): 1015–1021, 1995].

How can ostial obstruction be reduced?

Decongestants administered orally or in nasal sprays, and corticosteroids administered in nasal sprays can decrease mucosal swelling and edema to reduce ostial obstruction.

What is the major problem with decongestant nasal sprays?

When used for more than 3 to 4 days, the mucosa becomes accustomed to the effect of the decongestant, and there can be a significant rebound effect when the spray is discontinued. The rebound effect is characterized by severe nasal mucosal swelling and edema, which is very uncomfortable to the patient and which is relieved by administration of the decongestant spray. This physical "addiction" leads to repetitive or prolonged use of the decongestant spray.

When is a surgical consultation for a drainage procedure indicated?

In the case of recurrent or persistent sinusitis despite use of appropriate antibiotics

Helpful hints:

The color and character of the nasal discharge have traditionally been used to distinguish viral from bacterial infection; a thick green discharge is assumed to indicate a bacterial infection. However, respiratory mucus acquires the green color from the presence of polymorphonuclear neutrophil leukocytes (PMNs), not from bacteria. Even though PMNs tend to be more plentiful with bacterial infections, they are not exclusive to bacterial infections. Therefore, the assumption that a green discharge indicates a bacterial infection may not be valid.

PNEUMONIA

What is it?

An infectious disease that involves the parenchyma and alveoli of the lung. [Note: This discussion is limited to community-acquired pneumonia, which is the form most relevant to outpatient medicine; hospital-acquired (nosocomial) pneumonia is not covered.]

What are the common causes of pneumonia?

Viruses and bacteria

What bacteria commonly cause pneumonia?

Streptococcus pneumoniae (pneumococcus)
Other *Streptococcus* species
Mycoplasma pneumoniae
Haemophilus influenzae

Staphylococcus aureus
Legionella pneumophila
Mycobacterium tuberculosis
Chlamydia pneumoniae

Which bacteria is commonly found in patients with worsening symptoms after a recent viral pneumonia (post-viral bacterial pneumonia)?

Staphylococcus aureus

What are risk factors for pneumonia?

Advanced age (>65 years)
Immune compromise
Chronic lung disease
Significant underlying illness (e.g., diabetes mellitus)
Smoking
Household or occupational contacts with certain types of infections (e.g., *M. tuberculosis*)

What are the common signs and symptoms of pneumonia?

Productive cough
Malaise
Dyspnea
Fever
Rhonchi or crackles on lung examination (especially if findings are localized to one area of the lung)

What tests are used to diagnose pneumonia?

Chest x-ray is the test most commonly used to confirm the clinical assessment. Sputum Gram stain and culture do not usually provide information useful for diagnosis or treatment (with the possible exception of *M. tuberculosis* pneumonia). CBC with differential, serum electrolytes, urea nitrogen and creatinine, O_2 sat, and ABGs can help determine the severity of the infection and respiratory compromise. Tuberculin skin test (see Chapter 2) and serum antibody tests may be helpful in specific situations.

How is pneumonia treated?

Antibiotics
Supportive care when needed (oxygen, fluids, etc.)

What are first- and second-line antibiotics for pneumonia?

First line—penicillin, amoxicillin, erythromycin

Second line—amoxicillin/clavulanate, clarithromycin, second- or third-generation cephalosporins

How can some types of pneumonia be prevented?

Vaccination

For which organisms are effective vaccines available, and how often should they be administered?

Streptococcus pneumoniae—every 6 to 10 years

Influenza A and B—yearly

Who should be vaccinated?

High-risk persons (see above) should receive both pneumococcal and influenza vaccines.

Health care workers and close household contacts of high-risk persons should receive influenza vaccine yearly.

What are the admission criteria?

1. High-risk patients (see above), because of the risk of complications
2. Patients with evidence of significant respiratory compromise
3. Patients with significant dehydration
4. Patients who are unable to take oral medication (e.g., because of nausea or vomiting)
5. Patients who are unresponsive to outpatient therapy
6. Patients with inadequate resources at home (e.g., those who lack a phone or who do not have transportation to the hospital)
7. Patients with questionable treatment compliance or follow-up
8. Patients who have hemodynamic instability

CHRONIC OBSTRUCTIVE PULMONARY DISEASE (COPD)

What is it?

A chronic pulmonary process characterized by excessive bronchial secretions, bronchial hyperreactivity, and alveolar destruction. There is a continuum of disease ranging from mostly bronchial pathology (chronic bronchitis) on one end to mostly alveolar pathology (emphysema) on the other. Most patients have some combination of both.

What is the primary cause of COPD?

Smoking (80%–90% of patients)

What are other causes of COPD?

α-1 protease inhibitor deficiency (homozygous state)
Air pollution
Occupational exposure to chemical fumes or biologically inactive dusts

What are the common signs and symptoms of COPD?

    Mild to moderate disease:

Chronic nonpurulent sputum production
Dyspnea (especially with activity)
Wheezing
Distant heart sounds and barrel-shaped chest

    Severe disease:

Weight loss
Jugular venous distention
Use of accessory muscles of respiration

What are common diagnostic tests used in patients with COPD?

Pulmonary function tests (PFTs)
Chest x-rays
O_2 sat
ABGs

What are common findings on PFTs in patients with COPD?

Decreased forced expiratory volume in 1 second (FEV_1) and forced vital capacity with increased total capacity and residual volume

What are common findings on chest x-ray in patients with COPD?

Hyperexpanded lungs with increased anterior–posterior diameter of the chest, flattened diaphragm, and (sometimes) bullae

What finding on ABGs is characteristic of COPD?

A compensated respiratory acidosis with a mildly lowered pH, an elevated Pco_2, low Po_2, and elevated HCO_3

How is COPD treated?

Smoking cessation
Inhaled ipratropium

Inhaled β-agonists
Corticosteroids
Theophylline
Antibiotics
Low flow oxygen (2–4 L/min via nasal
cannula)

**Are antibiotics used in
patients with acute
exacerbations of COPD
that are not related to
infection?**

Yes

Why?

Patients improve more quickly if
antibiotic therapy is used. The
mechanism of this clinical phenomenon
is unclear.

**How does chronic
hypercarbia affect the
respiratory center in
patients with COPD?**

The respiratory center becomes less
responsive to elevations in P_{CO_2} that
normally drives it. The respiratory center
then becomes stimulated by hypoxia
rather than hypercarbia.

**How does this change in
respiratory stimulation
affect therapy for COPD?**

Oxygen must be administered at low
flow rates and the patient carefully
observed. Too much oxygen will
eliminate the hypoxic respiratory drive
(which the respiratory center needs) and
can lead to apnea.

**What are complications of
COPD?**

Pulmonary hypertension
Right ventricular hypertrophy
Cor pulmonale
Respiratory failure
Death

**What are the admission
criteria?**

1. Symptoms that do not respond
   quickly to high-dose inhaled
   ipratropium and β-agonists
2. Impending respiratory failure
3. Exacerbation associated with a
   significant infection (e.g., pneumonia)
4. Hemodynamic compromise

Helpful hints:

1. Smoking cessation is key if the
   destructive process is to be arrested.

It will not restore already damaged tissue but will prevent further destruction.

2. Advanced directives are extremely important in patients with worsening COPD. These patients need to know the risks and benefits of mechanical ventilation, especially as it pertains to the severity of their disease and the possibility that they may not be able to be weaned from the ventilator.

17   Common Skin Problems

What is it?	A spectrum of skin abnormalities characterized by comedones, papules, pustules, and cystic lesions of the skin of the face and upper back
What causes it?	Occlusion of the openings of the glands that produce sebum for the skin, increased sebum production, and overgrowth of bacteria (especially the acne bacillus, *Propionibacterium acnes*) results in accumulation of the sebum in the subcutaneous tissue and formation of papules and pustules. Destruction of the glands from swelling and inflammation leads to the formation of cysts.
In what age-group is acne most prevalent?	Adolescents
Why?	Androgen production during adolescence results in increased production of sebum. Acne is also more prevalent in males owing to their greater androgen production.
What are the signs and symptoms of acne?	Patients complain of blemishes on the face that are usually not painful. The lesions are papules with black or white hardened sebum occluding the pore (black or white comedones); inflamed pustules; or inflamed and often disfiguring cysts. The lesions are most often found on the face and/or trunk.

241

How is acne treated?   Specific treatment is directed toward the type of lesion found. General measures include frequent skin cleansing and avoidance of makeup and topical moisturizers. Food restriction (e.g., avoiding chocolate) has not been found to be useful in study populations. However, some individuals may notice worsening of acne with specific foods, which can then be avoided.

How are comedones treated?   Topical benzoyl peroxide
Topical tretinoin

How are pustules treated?   Topical antibiotics (erythromycin or clindamycin lotions or gels)
Systemic antibiotics (tetracycline is the antibiotic most frequently used)

How is cystic acne treated?   Systemic isotretinoin
Intralesion injection of steroids

What are some of the precautions employed when using isotretinoin?
- Women should not be pregnant and should use a reliable method of birth control (some recommend two methods) while using isotretinoin, because there is a high incidence of birth defects associated with its use.
- Serum lipids and liver enzymes should be followed every 2–4 weeks during treatment because of potential elevations associated with isotretinoin therapy.

Helpful hints:
1. Treatment will usually make the acne worse before it improves. Tell the patient to expect this and to continue using the medication. Give each medication change at least 4 weeks before re-evaluating for improvement.
2. Sunlight helps improve acne, so symptoms are usually better in the summer.
3. Excessive acne in an adolescent may be a sign of androgenic steroid use.

ATOPIC DERMATITIS (ECZEMA)

What is it?	An inflammatory condition of the skin related to atopy (allergy)
What other conditions are associated with atopic dermatitis?	Allergic rhinitis Asthma
What causes atopic dermatitis?	There is a genetic predisposition with variable penetrance. How the genetic predisposition influences the manifestations of disease is unclear.
What are the signs and symptoms of atopic dermatitis?	Itching and rash are the most common complaints. The skin is usually dry with areas of scaling and/or excoriation. These areas can be focal patches (nummular eczema), discrete parts of the body (e.g., the hands), or large and diffuse. Persons with heavily pigmented skin often have areas of variable pigment secondary to the inflammation. Common areas of involvement are the posterior aspect of the neck and flexor surfaces over joints (e.g., volar aspect of the elbow, behind the knee). Symptoms often are worse during particular seasons of the year.
How is atopic dermatitis treated?	Moisturization Antihistamines Topical steroids
How is the skin moisturized?	Frequent application of moisturizing lotions Avoidance of soaps that dry the skin (use oatmeal colloidal soap or Dove™ soap) Use of bath oil Avoidance of excessive bathing Application of petrolatum
How are antihistamines helpful?	They decrease itching. This helps to break the "scratch/itch cycle" that leads to an escalation of the pruritus and inflammation.

What is the role of topical steroids?

They decrease inflammation and usually help the lesions resolve. The lowest potency steroid that will help symptoms should be used. Overuse can lead to thinning of the skin and pigment changes. These side effects are most pronounced in the skin of the face; therefore, fluorinated steroids (higher potency) should be avoided on the face.

Helpful hints:

1. The question of whether to use warm water or cool water for washing and/ or bathing is still unanswered. Advise patients to use water at a temperature that doesn't worsen their symptoms.
2. Anticipate seasonal symptoms. Begin the moisturization program prior to any season that has been identified as troublesome for the patient.

IMPETIGO

What is it?

A superficial bacterial infection of the skin

What causes impetigo?

Usually, a small break in the integrity of the skin allows the penetration of bacteria.

What bacteria cause impetigo?

Group A streptococci and *Staphylococcus aureus*

What are the signs and symptoms of impetigo?

Mild to moderate itching
Erythematous patches with a honey-colored crust overlying the lesion (vesiculopustular impetigo), or bullous lesions (bullous impetigo)

How is impetigo treated?

Local care (soaking and cleansing the lesion with soap and water)
Topical mupirocin ointment
Systemic antibiotics (cephalexin)

Helpful hint:

Impetigo can be associated with the development of nephritis several weeks after the initial impetigo infection. Unfortunately, treatment does not prevent this complication.

CELLULITIS

What is it?	A bacterial infection that involves the entire thickness of the skin
What causes cellulitis?	Usually, a break in the skin allows the penetration of the bacteria that begin and sustain the infection. Persons with impairment of circulation and/or immunity are more susceptible to developing cellulitis.
What is the most common site of cellulitis?	The lower extremity
What bacterias cause cellulitis?	Many types. The most common causative organism is group A β-hemolytic streptococci (GABHS). Other streptococci and staphylococci are less common causes. Aerobic gram-negative enteric bacilli can also be involved; this is more likely in patients with predisposing conditions (e.g., diabetic foot ulcers).
What are the signs and symptoms of cellulitis?	Pain, tenderness, warmth, induration, and marked erythema of the involved skin. The border of the lesion is usually indistinct. Fever, chills, nausea, and headache are some of the systemic symptoms that can occur.
How is cellulitis treated?	Systemic antibiotics—oral or parenteral, depending on the severity of the process. Parenteral antibiotics are used in all patients deemed ill enough for admission to the hospital (see admission criteria on p. 246).
What are the antibiotics most commonly used to treat mild to moderate cellulitis on an outpatient basis?	Dicloxacillin Cephalexin
What is the most common serious complication of cellulitis?	Sepsis

Helpful hints:	During the initial examination, draw a line on the skin around the edge of the involved area so that progression or regression can be readily documented.
What are the admission criteria?	1. Large area of involvement 2. High fever and/or shaking chills 3. Significant underlying illness (e.g., diabetes mellitus, neutropenia) 4. Mental status changes 5. Nausea/vomiting precluding administration of oral antibiotics

CONTACT DERMATITIS

What is it?	An inflammatory response of the skin caused by contact of the skin with an offending substance
What causes contact dermatitis?	Allergy (type IV hypersensitivity response) Irritants (e.g., soaps, chemicals)
What are the substances that most commonly cause contact dermatitis?	Plant resins (e.g., poison ivy)
What are other common causes of contact dermatitis?	Topical antibiotics, cosmetics, soaps, detergents, and substances used in the clothing manufacturing process
When does contact dermatitis most commonly occur?	Spring and summer
Why?	The leaves of the plants that produce the resins are present to provide a contact surface for the skin. People are also outdoors more during spring and summer, and wearing less clothing.
What are the signs and symptoms of contact dermatitis?	Itching (usually intense) Erythema Small vesicles and areas of ruptured vesicles oozing clear fluid that are often found in a linear pattern on skin exposed to the causative substance

Can contact dermatitis be spread to other persons or other parts of the body from contact with the clear fluid that oozes from some lesions?	No. Once the resin has been removed from the skin by bathing, the rash cannot be spread to other areas of the body or other persons.
How is contact dermatitis treated?	Identification and removal/avoidance of the offending agent Antihistamines—decrease itching Topical corticosteroids—if only small areas of rash are present Systemic corticosteroids—for large areas of involvement and/or facial involvement
How long should oral corticosteroids be continued when treating contact dermatitis?	Most physicians recommend giving a tapering dose over 2 to 3 weeks. (This issue has not been addressed in a good randomized, controlled trial.)
Why this length of time?	To prevent a recurrence of the rash, which sometimes happens when a shorter treatment period is used
Helpful hints:	1. Plant resins can be carried on the fur of pets and transmitted to people. 2. The resin can be vaporized if the plant is burned and cause a rash on skin exposed to the smoke (usually the face and neck).

WARTS

This section excludes any information or reference to genital warts (see Chapter 9).

What are they?	Round or oval lesions of hyperkeratotic skin that have irregular surfaces which either protrude from the surrounding skin (warts on the hand) or penetrate into the surrounding skin (warts on the feet). Warts on the feet often have small (1–2 mm) black flecks scattered in the base of the lesion.
What causes warts?	A viral infection of the skin causes localized proliferation of the skin that

leads to the characteristic lesion. The hyperkeratotic lesion provides a nidus for the virus. Limited blood flow to the nidus protects the virus from exposure to and destruction by the immune system.

What is the term for warts on the plantar surface of the foot?

Plantar warts

What is the term used for warts in other locations on the skin?

Verrucous warts

Where are warts most commonly located?

The most common location is on the hand, but warts can occur in other locations on the body.

For what type of warts do patients most often seek medical attention?

Cosmetically unacceptable warts from 3 to 10 mm in diameter
Painful warts (plantar warts)

Why are plantar warts painful?

Plantar warts often cause pain from the pressure of walking or standing on the area of hypertrophied skin.

How are warts treated?

Cryotherapy (freezing)
Electrodesiccation
Excision
Application of acids (salicylic acid, bichloracetic acid, etc.)

What is the goal of therapy?

Destruction of the thickened, hyperkeratotic skin surrounding the virus

Why?

This allows the immune system to recognize and destroy the virus. The surrounding skin can then return to its normal thickness and contour.

What is the main complication of therapy?

Overaggressive use of the therapeutic modality can lead to scarring of the skin and permanent disfigurement. This can be a particularly difficult problem with plantar warts, because the scar tissue produces the same pain caused by the wart.

Is treatment of warts necessary?	No. Most warts will regress without treatment. However, most people prefer treatment for unsightly or painful warts.

TINEA

What is it?	A superficial skin infection and inflammation caused by dermatophytes, fungi that invade only keratinized tissues (skin, nails, and hair)
What are the terms used for tinea of the:	
Scalp?	Tinea capitis
Body?	Tinea corporis
Scrotum and inguinal area?	Tinea cruris
Nails?	Tinea unguium
Feet?	Tinea pedis
What are the most common dermatophytes?	*Trichophyton, Epidermophyton,* and *Microsporum*
What are the signs and symptoms of tinea?	Itching, flaking/scaling, and erythema are common to all types of tinea. Pustular lesions of the scalp, thickened/discolored nails, hyper- or hypopigmentation of the skin, and annular lesions of the skin with central clearing are common findings in specific areas of involvement.
What diagnostic tests are used to confirm fungal infections?	Skin, scalp, or nail scrapings mixed with 10% potassium hydroxide (KOH) and examined under the high power of the microscope for fungal organisms (see Chapter 2) Skin, scalp, or nail scrapings sent for culture
How are cutaneous fungal infections treated?	Topical or systemic antifungal antibiotics (e.g., miconazole, ketoconazole)

Which types of tinea require systemic therapy, and how long should each be treated?	Tinea capitis: 1–3 months Tinea unguium: 3–12 months (depending on the agent used)
What parameters should be monitored when using systemic antifungal agents?	Liver function CBC
Helpful hints:	1. Examination of the scalp under a Wood's lamp is no longer helpful in diagnosis of tinea capitis because the organisms that fluoresce (*Microsporum*) are no longer a common cause of this infection. 2. Newer systemic antifungal agents (e.g., itraconazole) appear to be better at treating tinea unguium (shorter duration of treatment) but are very expensive. However, the cost difference is not so great when you consider the extended length of time the older agents need to be taken (up to 12 months), and the cost of monitoring the blood counts and liver enzymes during that extended period. 3. Antifungal agents are better absorbed from the GI tract if taken with fatty foods.

ACUTE URTICARIA (HIVES, ANGIOEDEMA)

What is urticaria?	The cutaneous manifestation of a type I hypersensitivity reaction (i.e, mediated by immunoglobulin E).
What causes urticaria?	Many diverse stimuli. The more common causes include medications, foods, insect stings (e.g., bee sting), and anxiety.
What are the signs and symptoms of urticaria?	Itching followed by wheals (small areas of blanching of the skin) that subsequently are surrounded by larger areas of erythema (flare). Lesions usually come and go, often in different locations. Swelling of the face, hands, tongue, and/or larynx can occur in more

	severe cases. Swelling of the larynx is usually associated with stridor.
How are urticaria treated?	Antihistamines (diphenhydramine, cetirizine) Subcutaneous epinephrine (Patients with known sensitivity to Hymenoptera—bees, wasps, and ants—should be given a pre-filled syringe of epinephrine to carry with them at all times.) Systemic corticosteroids
How are urticaria prevented?	Avoidance of offending agents (chemicals, foods, medications) Desensitization (Hymenoptera)
What is the potential serious complication of urticaria?	Anaphylaxis. Urticaria can be the initial manifestation of this more serious, systemic type I hypersensitivity reaction.
What are the clinical findings of anaphylaxis?	Laryngeal edema as evidenced by stridor, dyspnea, wheezing, tachypnea, tachycardia, hypotension, seizures, and/or cardiorespiratory collapse
How is anaphylaxis treated?	Anaphylaxis requires emergency medical treatment. Subcutaneous epinephrine, parenteral corticosteroids, and parenteral antihistamines are the medications administered initially. The patient should be transported to the nearest medical facility and followed in an intensive care unit. IV fluids, vasopressors (epinephrine or isoproterenol), and endotracheal intubation with mechanical ventilation may be required.
Helpful hints:	Urticaria can persist for months or years without identification of a definitive etiology. These chronic urticaria are not IgE mediated, tend to eventually resolve, and are not usually associated with anaphylaxis.

HERPES ZOSTER (SHINGLES)

What is it?	A painful dermatitis occurring in a dermatomal pattern

What is a dermatome?

An area of skin whose sensory input travels through a single dorsal root ganglia

What organism causes shingles?

Varicella-zoster virus

How?

After the initial varicella-zoster infection (chickenpox), the virus exists in a dormant state in the dorsal nerve root ganglia. The virus can reactivate along the dorsal (sensory) nerve and cause the dermatitis.

What causes reactivation of the virus?

The exact triggers are unknown, but conditions that cause impaired immunity (e.g., physical and emotional stress, illness, advanced age, HIV) are frequently associated with outbreaks.

What are the common signs and symptoms of shingles?

Painful patches of erythema with vesicles and small ulcerations that are unilateral (i.e., follow along a single dermatome). The trunk and face are the most common areas of involvement. Moderate to severe pain is one of the hallmarks of shingles. Occasionally, the pain precedes the outbreak of the rash.

How are shingles treated?

Analgesics
Antiviral agents (acyclovir, famciclovir)

What is the most troublesome complication of shingles?

Postherpetic neuralgia

Why?

The pain persists along the dermatome for weeks to months after the rash clears. The pain can be debilitating and difficult to treat.

Can postherpetic neuralgia be prevented?

No. Neuralgia associated with the acute episode can be shortened with antiviral therapy, but the duration of true postherpetic neuralgia is unaffected by any therapy.

How is postherpetic neuralgia treated?

Analgesics
Topical capsaicin cream
Regional nerve blocks
Tricyclic antidepressants

Helpful hints:

1. Recurrent episodes or involvement of multiple dermatomes may indicate a more serious problem with immunity, such as HIV or malignancy. Further evaluation is indicated.
2. Postherpetic neuralgia is more common in older patients.

18

Evidence-Based
Medicine (EBM)

**What is evidence-based
medicine (EBM)?**

An approach to medical care that
emphasizes the use of the best available
evidence to make evaluation and
treatment decisions. In contrast,
traditional medicine emphasizes
pathophysiology and anecdote.

**What is the basis of
treatment strategies in:**

    EBM?

The best EBM treatment strategies are
based on randomized controlled trials
(RCTs) that demonstrate improved
patient outcomes.

    Traditional medicine?

Treatment strategies are grounded in
inductive reasoning based on the present
state of understanding of the
pathophysiology of a disease or an
anecdotal observation in treating one or
more patients.

**In considering the
question of using
medication to lower
cholesterol, describe the
approach taken by:**

    Traditional medicine

Observation—Elevated cholesterol is
associated with increased risk of
myocardial infarction (MI).
Inductive reasoning—If elevated
cholesterol is associated with MI,
lowering the cholesterol with
medication must be helpful.
Result—Drugs that lower cholesterol are
used extensively and assumed to
decrease the risk of MI.

EBM	*Observation*—Drugs that lower cholesterol are used extensively and assumed to decrease the risk of MI. *Question*—What are the objective outcomes (as opposed to the anecdotal observations) of patients who take these medications? (Do patients who take cholesterol lowering agents live longer? Do they have fewer myocardial infarctions? Do they stay in the hospital fewer days? Do they have fewer procedures?) *Evidence-based answer*—Some medications do nothing, some seem to be harmful, and some seem to be helpful. *Deductive reasoning*—Choose an agent that has been shown to be helpful in a population that is most like the patient for whom the medication is being prescribed.
Are the two approaches mutually exclusive?	No—EBM is merely the next logical step from traditional medicine. Pathophysiology and clinical observation (traditional medicine) are the basis for developing new treatment strategies that can then be tested in RCTs to document improved outcomes. EBM incorporates the results of these studies into treatment decisions.
What is the danger, in traditional medicine, of untested clinical observation (anecdotal information)?	Traditional medicine is extremely susceptible to multiple biases and invalid logic. One should always be skeptical of anecdotal information, even if presented by a respected expert. Evidence suggests that experts are as susceptible as anyone else to bias and invalid logic.
What are POEMs?	Patient Oriented Outcomes that Matter—the focus of EBM.
Give some examples.	Mortality Morbidity Complications Cost Time lost from work

(For example, patients don't care if their cholesterol is high, but they want to avoid having an MI because they don't want to die, be disabled, lose time from work, or be in the hospital.)

What are the three steps for incorporating EBM into practice?

1. Obtaining relevant information
2. Evaluating the validity of the information obtained
3. Initiating information-based change into practice

How does one efficiently sort through the available information to obtain that which is relevant?

Usefulness is proportional to relevance and validity of the information, and inversely proportional to the work needed to acquire the information, as described in the following formula:

$$\text{Usefulness} = \frac{\text{Relevance} \times \text{Validity}}{\text{Work}}$$

Look for POEMs that are common to your practice and will change what you do (Relevance). Reading studies that don't look at outcomes in an appropriate format (RCT) or that don't apply to common problems in your practice can waste valuable time (Work). As the formula above shows, increasing relevance and decreasing work increases the usefulness of the information.

Why is it important to assess the validity of the information obtained?

If a study is not valid, usefulness is zero.

How does one assess the validity of a study?

If you are not comfortable with your ability to critically review a study for validity, you must learn the skill or find someone who can do it for you. Several journals have sections devoted to critically reviewing studies that affect practice (Journal of Family Practice Journal Club, American College of Physicians Journal Club, and Evidence-Based Medicine).

Why is it important to initiate changes in practice based on POEMs?	It would be unethical to have the ability to improve your patients' outcomes and not implement that strategy into your practice.
Why have changes in medical practice occurred so slowly?	Most physicians don't know the difference between POEMs and DOEs—Disease-Oriented Evidence, or pathophysiology—and/or are unable to critically review a study for validity. Therefore, most physicians don't know which data are important and which are incomplete.
Are practice guidelines a good way to implement EBM?	Maybe. Some practice guidelines are excellent sources of EBM and some are not.
What are the two main types of practice guidelines?	Evidence-Based Guidelines Consensus Guidelines
How is an Evidence-Based Guideline developed?	The panel developing the guideline extensively searches and reviews all of the world's literature on a given topic. It then develops a guideline based on the best available evidence (Table 18–1).
How are Consensus-Based Guidelines developed?	Consensus-Based Guidelines are developed by convening experts in a particular field and asking them to come to a consensus on recommendations for a particular clinical situation. The American Cancer Society guidelines are developed in this manner.

Table 18-1. Development of Evidence-Based Guidelines: US Preventive Health Task Force Guide to Clinical Preventive Services

Step 1. The US Preventive Health Task Force reviewed all the available literature for screening strategies available for preventive health services.

Step 2. The quality of evidence was ranked in decreasing order of reliability: randomized controlled trial, nonrandomized controlled trial, cohort studies, case-control studies, uncontrolled experiments, descriptive studies, and expert opinion.

Step 3. Each test was then rated A, B, C, D, or E, depending on its usefulness as a screening tool for the disease for which it was studied.

Result—an excellent evidenced-based guideline that clinicians can use to focus their preventive health

What is the problem with Consensus-Based Guidelines?

Consensus-Based Guidelines are fraught with bias and can be dominated by one or two outspoken persons. Guidelines developed in this manner can end up as a poor representation of the available evidence.

How should the primary care physician approach practice guidelines?

Use caution. Read more than just the recommendations. It is imperative that you know the methods used to develop the guideline before implementing it in your practice. Guidelines may have a low Work factor, but if they are not Valid, their usefulness is zero.

Helpful hints:

Several resources for more information on EBM and the patient-centered approach to clinical decision making:

1. Shaughnessy AF: Becoming an information master: a guidebook to the medical information jungle. *J Fam Pract* 39(5), 489–499, 1994.
2. Slawson DC: Becoming a medical information master: feeling good about not knowing everything. *J Fam Pract* 38(5), 505–513, 1994.
3. U.S. Task Force: Introduction. In *Guide to Clinical Preventive Services: Report of the US Preventive Services Task Force,* 2nd ed. Baltimore: Williams & Wilkins, 1996.

Index

Note: Page numbers in *italic* indicate illustrations; page numbers followed by t indicate tables.